ADVANCE PRAISE

"This book is an amazing resource for parents bringing home a newborn baby. It answers many of the common questions new parents have and it also explains many medical issues in a thorough and easy to understand way. An excellent quick read to put parents' minds at ease."
—Neelesh Kenia, M.D., F.A.A.P., Pediatrician, San Francisco, CA

"Dr. Jung brings a wealth of common-sense, no-nonsense advice to soon-to-be parents. His writing style is conversational, easy to understand, and humorous. The advice offered was gathered over his years of practice and will be invaluable to patients."
—Robert Yetman, M.D., F.A.A.P., Pediatrician in Houston, TX

"I would be thrilled if expectant and new parents read this book! This guide will definitely elevate the quality of the interaction between the pediatric provider and parent, paving the way for more effective visits and better exchange of information."
—Rakesh Chopra, M.D., F.A.A.P., Lead Physician of Chopra Pediatrics in Altoona, PA

"Thorough yet concise, Dr. Jung's new book provides new parents the peace of mind they need."
—Suny Liaw, M.D., F.A.A.P., Instructor in Pediatrics at Harvard Medical School

"A great overview of the most common questions all new parents have. Almost like having your pediatrician sitting on the bookshelf!"
—Mark D. Hormann, M.D., F.A.A.P., Pediatrician in Houston, TX

"*What to Know Before Having Your Baby* is an intelligent, humorous, concise, and reassuring guide that will be at the top of my suggested reading list for new parents in my pediatric practice."
—Adrian Clarke, M.D., F.A.A.P., Pediatrician in Dallas, TX

"There are two types of EBM: evidence-based medicine and experience-based medicine. This book has both. Written by a seasoned pediatrician and father, parents will find it filled with advice regarding the care of their newborn that is scientifically sound and everyday practical."
—Mark Ward M.D., F.A.A.P., Director of the Pediatric Residency Program at Texas Children's Hospital in Houston, TX

ADVANCE PRAISE

What to Know Before Having Your Baby

An Illustrated Guide

Peter Jung, M.D.

Illustrations by Becky Seo Kim

What to Know Before Having Your Baby

Library of Congress Cataloging-in-Publication Data is available upon request.
ISBN 978-1-57826-664-7

All Hatherleigh Press titles are available for bulk purchase, special promotions, and premiums. For information about reselling and special purchase opportunities, please call 1-800-528-2550 and ask for the Special Sales Manager.

Cover and Interior Design by Carolyn Kasper

10 9 8 7 6 5 4 3 2 1
Printed in the United States

Contents

Introduction

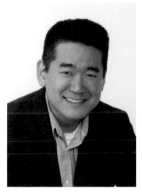

THERE IS NOTHING that brings greater joy than having a baby. But then come all the questions.

When I first started practicing pediatrics in 2002, the first thing I worked on was creating a "newborn booklet" to address questions frequently asked by new parents. It started off as a flimsy pamphlet with just under 10 pages of "advice" from a neophyte pediatrician. Since then, I have gained a wealth of experience as a doctor, encountered myriads of differing feeding and sleeping philosophies for babies, and, most importantly, raised three children of my own. Along the way, that flimsy pamphlet grew to nearly 50 pages and has become what many of my patients call their "newborn Bible."

Every doctor at Blue Fish Pediatrics has contributed their own take on snot, fevers, and colic, but none has been more influential than my original partner, Dr. William Pielop. In the early days of Blue Fish, we would trade aphorisms and workshop spiels at lunch, trying to figure out just the right way to explain how to feed a newborn baby to an anxious new mom.

This second book was born from those many lunch conversations and owes a lot to the Blue Fish newborn book. Hopefully, it will serve to assuage your anxiety about the many rashes, habits, and bodily findings that you will encounter as you raise your baby. The vast majority of things that parents observe are what we call "normal abnormals"—findings that are not a true health concern, but which prompt a parent to wonder, "Does this need to be evaluated?"

This book will cover the common questions that so often cause unnecessary worry for new parents. The answers to these questions, along with the accompanying pictures and short vignettes, are intended to help reassure moms and dads that their baby is healthy *and* give them peace of mind. However, as with my first book, the information here is not intended to replace your doctor. Rather, it is meant to enhance the conversations you have with your doctor so that each check-up can be more efficient and productive. If you suspect that there *is* a serious problem with your newborn, parents are encouraged to seek medical advice from their pediatrician.

I hope that this book will help bring peace of mind, and answer many of your concerns so that you can fully enjoy every precious moment with your newborn.

—Peter Y. Jung, M.D., F.A.A.P.

Chapter 1

DELIVERY DAY

WHEN THE day finally comes to deliver your baby, it may feel like you are suddenly living inside a whirlwind of questions, tests, prodding, and probing. But when it is all said and done, and you are finally holding your newborn in your arms, everything in the world will feel just right.

But then comes another barrage of questions, tests, prodding, and probing! Except, this time, it is for your baby. Vitamin K, prophylactic eye antibiotics, newborn screens, and jaundice tests are just some of the many tests that will be offered as options to you and your newborn. In general, it is safest to default to accepting any of the hospital screens that are offered to you. Most of these protocols have been put in place for a reason, and there is almost always solid medical evidence supporting their use.

Of course, it is always more comforting to understand *why* these tests are being recommended. Although it may feel intrusive, and you may empathize with the pain your baby goes through, your newborn *will* benefit from each of the measures taken. And rest assured—they will retain no long term memory of any of the needles and injections.

APGAR

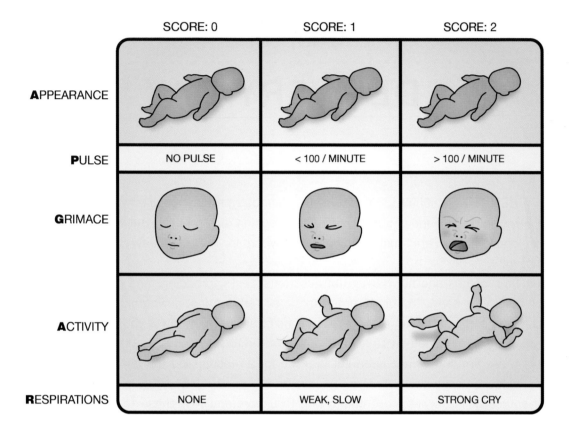

	SCORE: 0	SCORE: 1	SCORE: 2
APPEARANCE			
PULSE	NO PULSE	< 100 / MINUTE	> 100 / MINUTE
GRIMACE			
ACTIVITY			
RESPIRATIONS	NONE	WEAK, SLOW	STRONG CRY

The **APGAR score** is a number given to newborn babies soon after they are born—specifically, at the 1 minute and 5 minute mark—which measures an infant's general state of well-being along five subjective metrics: the baby's general **A**ppearance; their **P**ulse; their facial expression, and whether or not they are **G**rimacing; their general level of **A**ctivity; and their rate of **R**espiration. A numerical rating of 0–2 is given for each category, up to a maximum score of 10.

The score was originally developed in 1952 by an anesthesiologist named Virginia Apgar. Although it was originally used to ascertain the effects of maternal anesthesia on babies, it is now commonly employed to determine whether there is an immediate need for the baby to receive extra medical care. The lower the score, the greater the need for intervention and for possible transfer to a Neonatal Intensive Care Unit (NICU).

There is only a weak correlation, if any, between an infant's APGAR score and their long-term developmental outcomes. The APGAR score is best utilized as a quick communication tool between caretakers in the first few days of life. Even then, other evaluative information (such as the physical exam and vital signs) are more essential, and ultimately more reliable.

NEWBORN SCREEN

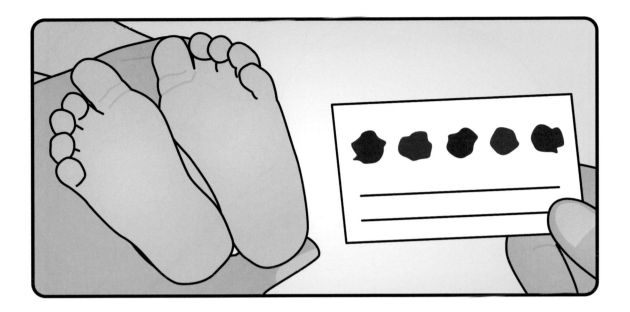

A **newborn screen** is a preliminary examination of the infant, typically completed in the first 1–2 weeks of life. Some states require only a single screen, while others require two screens (one immediately after birth, and a second one a week later). A health professional will take a few drops of blood from the heel and place it on a screening card to be sent for testing. Exactly what is tested for in the screening depends on the state; each state requires a different array of diseases to be tested for.

Newborn screens help detect dangerous diseases early in life, especially those that may not show any signs until the damage has already occurred. These conditions can lead to serious problems such as brain damage, organ damage, and even death. If detected early enough, the infant can receive proper treatment and avoid serious complications from these relatively rare conditions.

A word to the wise: newborn screen tests are often calibrated to be *extremely* sensitive, leading to many false positives. The logic is that the state would much rather have too many tests return false positives, as opposed to risking a single false negative test—a scenario where a true illness is missed by the newborn screen. In other words, a positive test does not *necessarily* mean a true disease is present. Follow-up studies and medical consultation can confirm whether a true problem exists and ascertain what treatment is available.

EYE ANTIBIOTIC OINTMENT

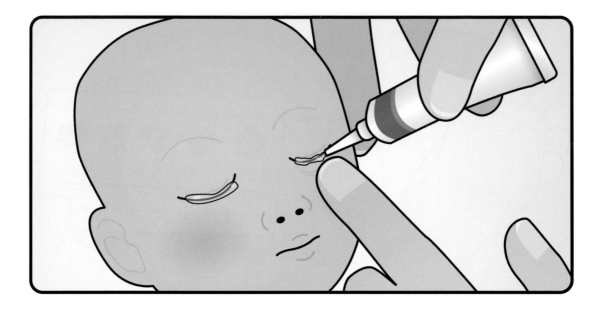

Soon after your baby is born, they will likely have a clear antibiotic ointment placed on their eyes. This is to prevent an infection of the eyes called **ophthalmia neonatorum**, which is most commonly caused by the Gonorrhea and Chlamydia bacteria being present in the mother (as sexually transmitted diseases).

The risk of this infection is quite low, but in those cases where it does present, it has the potential to lead to blindness. Comparatively, the side effects of antibiotic ointment to the infant is minimal—most commonly, the child experiences a slight, short-lived irritation of the eyes. Most states have a law requiring that all infants receive this treatment as soon as they are born, regardless of the mother's risk of having these illnesses.

Vitamin K (2, 7, 9, 10, S, C)
Contact activation (intrinsic) pathway

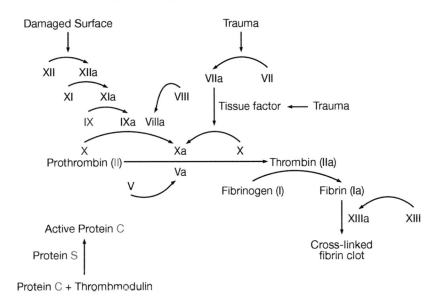

Vitamin K is a fat-soluble vitamin that is needed to make certain blood clotting factors in our body. Adults fulfill the majority of their vitamin K needs through the consumption of green leafy vegetables in their diet, with a smaller amount received via the production of the vitamin from healthy bacteria in our intestines.

Babies, on the other hand, are born with a very small amount of vitamin K in their body. As such, they benefit greatly from an injection (the preferred method in the United States) or oral supplementation on their first day of life. Consumption of vitamin K by the mother prior to birth is likely helpful to increase vitamin K storage in the baby; however, babies have a limited amount of fat and there is no evidence to support that increased intake by the mother alone is adequate to significantly improve a baby's vitamin K levels. The safest protection for your baby is to receive a vitamin K injection at time of birth, per routine hospital protocol.

Lack of vitamin K can lead to various clotting problems, the most serious being a bleed in the brain, which can result in death or long-term disabilities. This can happen anytime during the first 12 weeks of life and can occur even if the birth itself was non-traumatic. Other issues can arise when boys are circumcised and can lead to uncontrolled bleeding.

A last note: some parents reject vitamin K injections, largely based on a single study from the early 1990s, which found a possible link between intramuscular vitamin K administration and leukemia. Multiple studies since then have failed to confirm this finding.

VITAMIN D

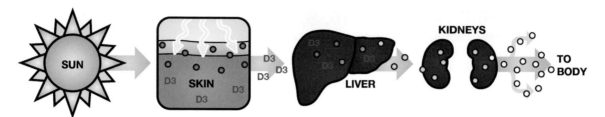

1. Ultraviolet-B rays convert a derivative of cholesterol – already present in the **skin** – into Vitamin D3, which then travels to the liver.

2. The **liver** converts Vitamin D3 to another form called 25-hydroxy-Vitamin D, which is what doctors measure in the blood.

3. The **kidneys** convert this form to the final active hormone that may have many effects throughout the body, including enabling calcium absorption in the intestines.

The American Academy of Pediatrics (AAP) currently recommends that all infants receive 400 IU of **vitamin D** per day. Vitamin D deficiency can possibly lead to rickets (a disease of weak bones) and other medical problems.

Infants can acquire vitamin D either through their diet or through exposure to sunlight. Studies show that babies who receive 10–30 minutes of sunlight per week (while wearing only a diaper) will likely produce all the vitamin D their body needs. Similarly, babies who receive 30 minutes to 2 hours of sunlight per week (fully clothed, with no hat) also are likely to produce all the vitamin D they need. Babies who do not receive adequate sunlight exposure and/or have dark skin are most at risk for vitamin D deficiency.

Because human milk only contains a vitamin D concentration of 25 IU per liter or less, the AAP recommends all breastfed babies receive a supplement of 400 IU per day. (Infant formulas are all fortified with vitamin D. In general, formula fed babies require little to no supplementation.) Over-the-counter brands of vitamin D containing 400 IU/ml or 400 IU/drop are readily available and easy to use. In babies who receive an adequate amount of sunlight, vitamin D supplementation may not be necessary; however, the current recommendation is that all breastfed babies receive vitamin D supplementation.

What to Know Before Having Your Baby

JAUNDICE

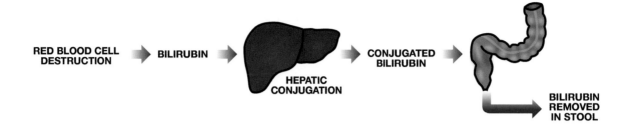

RED BLOOD CELL DESTRUCTION → BILIRUBIN → HEPATIC CONJUGATION → CONJUGATED BILIRUBIN → BILIRUBIN REMOVED IN STOOL

Almost all babies will display some level of yellowness (known as **jaundice**) in their first few days of life—especially breastfed babies. When red blood cells die, they naturally become a yellow waste product called **bilirubin**, which is then processed by the liver and disposed of in the stool. Because the baby's liver is not yet fully mature and cannot process bilirubin, it returns to the blood and eventually stains the eyes and skin yellow (temporarily).

Most infant jaundice will improve without any intervention; however, some children will require a little help. One of the best ways to help your infant break down the bilirubin in their system is exposure to sunlight. At home, you can place your baby in **indirect sunlight** with just a diaper on. This can be done inside the home next to a window, even on a cloudy day. Hold them in the light for 10–15 minutes at a time, three to four times a day.

If your child's jaundice is quite noticeable—if your child looks very yellow (almost fluorescent) or the whites of their eyes have turned noticeably yellow—they should be evaluated by a pediatrician. They may need to have their bilirubin level checked, and they may need to receive **phototherapy** (placing them under a blue ultraviolet light) either at home or in the hospital.

You may have heard that stopping breastfeeding will help jaundice. While it is true that breastfed babies are more likely to display jaundice, studies have clearly shown that there is little benefit to stopping breastfeeding for jaundice purposes.

Head Circumference
Birth to 5 years (percentiles)

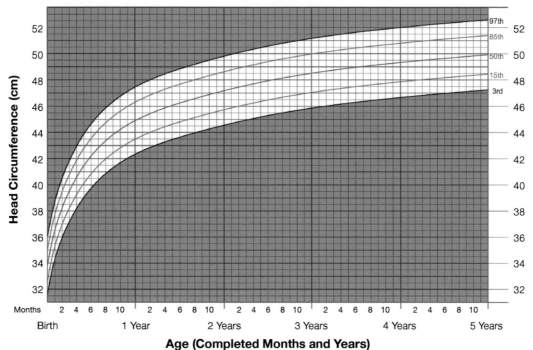

WHO Child Growth Standards

At each well child visit, your pediatrician will measure the circumference of your infant's head, comparing it against your infant's height and weight. Like any other growth parameter, your pediatrician will be more concerned with the *trend* of your infant's head circumference—also known as the **frontal-occipital circumference (FOC)**—than the actual percentile. Once a baby has been measured at 3–4 well child visits, a pattern will emerge with the FOC.

Parents often worry if their child's FOC is too small or too big, or mismatched with the percentiles of height and weight. Babies high on the weight and/or height curve can be low on the FOC curve; conversely, babies who are low on the weight and/or height curve can be high on the FOC curve. There is nothing to be concerned about with mismatched percentiles—bear in mind, the difference between the 25th percentile and the 75th percentile FOC for an infant is approximately 2 centimeters, which is an indiscernible amount for the naked eye.

As long as the FOC is tracking along a similar percentile curve each time, there is little to be worried about. If the FOC begins to cross the percentile curves, moving either up or down with a noticeable deviation, further evaluation will be necessary. Additionally, any baby with an FOC that is extremely large or small that is not consistent with the genetic pattern of the family may also require further evaluation.

WEIGHT LOSS AND CURVE

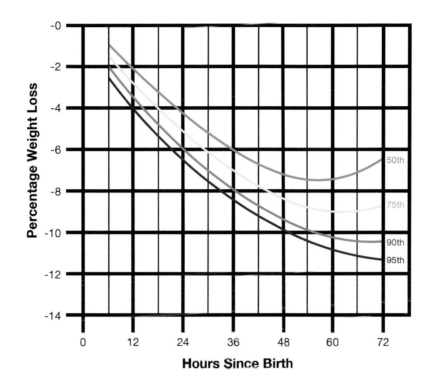

Nearly all babies will lose up to 10 percent of their body weight over their first 5–6 days of life. This is normal, and is rarely a cause for alarm. The major cause of this is a loss of fluids through evaporation from their waterlogged skin, urine output, and stool output. Additionally, most babies may need a few days before they are able to eat effectively, as there is an initial learning curve (and they are quite sleepy when born).

It is highly atypical for a baby's weight loss to become so severe that hospitalization is necessary. As a rule of thumb, after hitting the lowest point of their weight which is usually around the 5th day of life, babies should regain about 0.5–1 ounce of weight per day. Most babies will get back to their birth weight by 10–14 days of age. However, some breastfed babies may take a bit longer.

Typically, formula-fed babies will regain weight faster than breastfed babies, as the learning curve for bottle-feeding is quicker than breastfeeding, and there is never a supply issue. Some moms need a few days (to have a good letdown effect) before they can adequately produce enough breast milk to match their baby's needs.

Overall, as long as the weight trend is healthy and the baby is eating approximately eight times a day, there is little cause for concern. Regular weight checks at the pediatrician's office can alleviate any concerns parents may have.

TAKE-HOME POINTS

★ APGAR scores are helpful for relaying information right at birth, but have a weak correlation to long-term development.

★ State mandated newborn screen tests can help detect rare diseases at birth so that affected children can receive proper treatment in a timely fashion.

★ The risk of an eye infection is quite low at birth, but because it has been proven to be safe and the consequences of an infection can be severe, antibiotic ointment should always be used prophylactically.

★ Any baby can be vitamin K deficient at birth, which can lead to serious bleeding issues. As such, vitamin K should always be given prophylactically.

★ Most children will receive all the vitamin D they need from small amounts of sun exposure, but for breastfed babies, a supplement may be helpful.

★ Jaundice is very common and most babies will improve without intervention; however, if they look fluorescent yellow, they may benefit from phototherapy.

★ Head circumferences that are extremely large or small and which are not consistent with the genetic pattern of the family may require further evaluation. In general, the trend of the head circumference curve is more important than the actual percentile.

★ All babies will have some weight loss at birth, with most returning back to their birth weight by 10–14 days of age.

Chapter 2

SKIN

AFTER THE initial thrill of holding your newborn passes, the first thing parents tend to notice are all of the strange rashes and skin findings that appear on their new baby. This will evoke some anxiety and concern, but rest assured that most dermatologic issues at this age are fleeting. Often, no treatment is necessary; but at times—to help a rash disappear a bit sooner or to reduce discomfort—low-dose steroid creams, lotions, and a few other tricks can help manage the skin's issues.

Of course, as most issues are cosmetic only, it is also perfectly reasonable to let things run their course, and more often than not rashes will resolve on their own.

CRADLE CAP

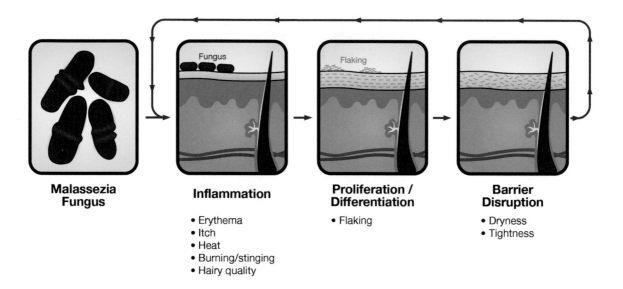

Malassezia Fungus

Inflammation
- Erythema
- Itch
- Heat
- Burning/stinging
- Hairy quality

Proliferation / Differentiation
- Flaking

Barrier Disruption
- Dryness
- Tightness

It is common for newborn babies to have white or yellow dandruff-like flakes on their scalps. This skin change is called "**cradle cap**" or seborrheic dermatitis. No one knows for sure why this happens, but the current theory is that it is related to oil production from our skin and a possible reaction to a fungus naturally found on the skin called Malessezia.

If the flakes become thick and scale-like, you can put baby oil on the scalp overnight and use a baby brush to remove them once they have softened in the morning. Adult anti-dandruff shampoos can be used daily or every other day to help keep the condition at bay. Do *not* get these shampoos in your baby's eyes, and be sure to do a thorough job rinsing all of the shampoo off your baby's skin, as they can be irritating.

After several days of use, try to use the shampoo less and less, and only for maintenance purposes. You also have the option not to treat at all, as cradle cap is a purely cosmetic issue which will resolve on its own with time (usually within the first few months of life).

ECZEMA

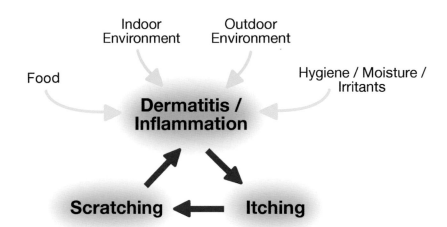

The term **eczema** refers to an inflammation of the skin leading to itching, redness, swelling, and peeling of the skin. This can happen for any number of reasons, including sensitivity to a particular thing in the environment, weather changes, certain foods, sensitivity to a lotion or clothing material, etc.

Almost all babies will have a small amount of eczema at some point in their life. Parents often worry that eczema will become chronic and severe, and while this *is* seen in a small percentage of children, most will outgrow any issues within the first two years of life, with flare-ups being small and easily manageable.

While eczema cannot be cured, it *can* be controlled in all but the severest of cases, until the child (hopefully) outgrows it.

Although some children will have specific triggers (such as dust, pollen or a certain food) that seem to elicit an eczema breakout, it is better to think of eczema as a general sensitivity of the skin. For example, an eczema-prone child who is sensitive to peanuts will almost certainly have eczema issues when exposed to peanuts; however, just because a family successfully avoids peanuts does not mean they will prevent all eczema exacerbations as there may be a host of other things in the environment that can also trigger the eczema.

ERYTHEMA TOXICUM

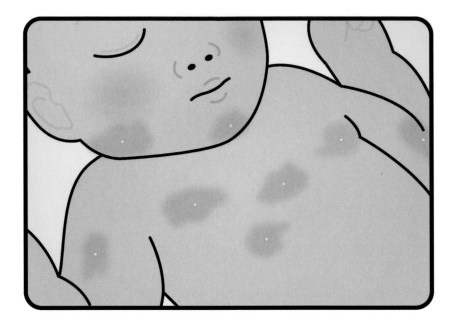

Erythema toxicum is a very common rash, usually seen in the first 1–2 days of an infant's life. It appears as scattered red splotches, with or without tiny yellowish-white bumps in the center of the lesion. They can appear anywhere on the body, including the face, trunk, arms, and legs.

No one is certain what causes erythema toxicum. The current theory is that it has to do with a reaction of the immune system; to what, we don't know. However, the rash is benign and does not require treatment; it will typically disappear by 1–2 weeks of life.

SEBACEOUS GLAND HYPERPLASIA

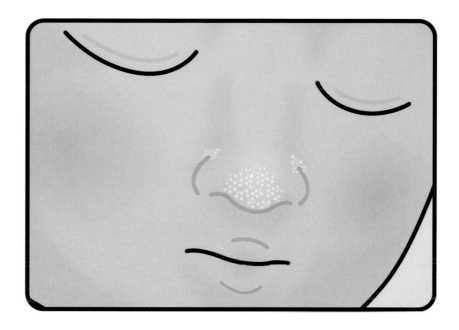

Some babies will have a large amount of yellowish-white dots on their noses called **sebaceous gland hyperplasia**. Sebum is an oily substance secreted by the sebaceous glands of the skin to help lubricate and waterproof the skin and hair. Hormones from the mother may stimulate these sebaceous glands to grow rapidly, giving the nose its characteristic appearance.

Sebaceous gland hyperplasia is benign and will go away without treatment; however, it can be helpful to wash the area with a mild soap once daily.

MILIA

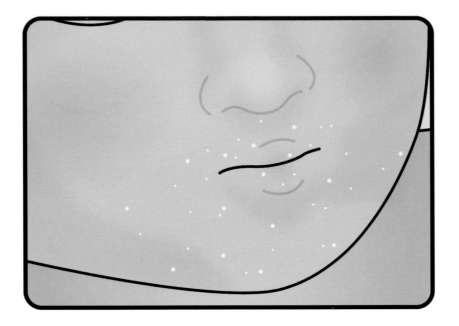

Some babies have small white dots on their nose, face, and other parts of their body called **milia**. Unlike sebaceous gland hyperplasia, these bumps are raised, and are not clustered together. Milia are essentially small cysts filled with skin debris; in other words, small bumps filled with a minute amount of trapped skin.

Milia will resolve on their own and do not need to be treated. It is recommended not to pop these lesions, as doing so may lead to an infection.

NEONATAL ACNE

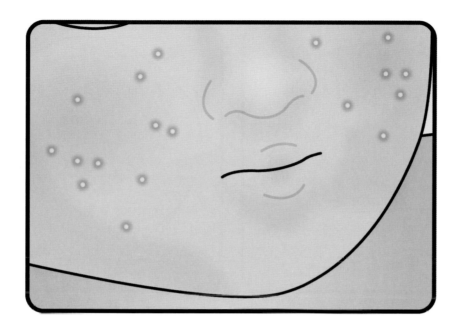

In the first few months of life, most babies will at some point develop a rash, usually starting on the cheeks, which can include the scalp, face, neck, upper back, upper torso, and ears. This condition is often called "**neonatal acne**," but has recently been renamed "**neonatal cephalic pustulosis**." Like cradle cap, it is thought to be an immune system response to the presence of a common fungus that naturally resides on the skin, called Malessezia.

Neonatal acne is also likely linked to an increased stimulation of the sebaceous glands brought on by the presence of the mother's hormones, resulting in an increased production of **sebum**. (Sebum is an oily substance secreted by the sebaceous glands to help lubricate and waterproof the skin and hair.)

Neonatal acne generally peaks at about 1 month of age and can last several months. The rash does not require treatment, but 1 percent hydrocortisone cream (sold over-the-counter) applied to the non-facial areas two times per day for about one week will reduce the amount of inflammation, especially behind the ears and around the neck. If used on the face, 0.5 percent hydrocortisone may be safer, though it should still be used sparingly, avoiding the area around the eyes.

NEVUS SIMPLEX

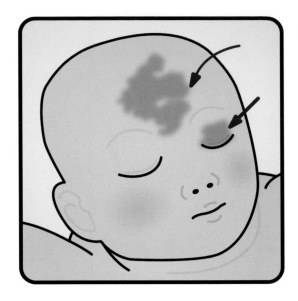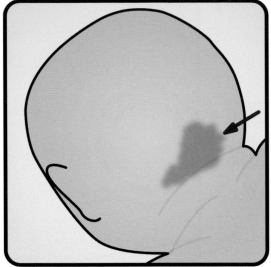

Nevus simplexes are normal pink-red patches seen on newborn infants, commonly found on the eyelids, the back of the neck, and in between the eyes. They are less commonly found on the scalp, nose, lips, and back. (A Nevus simplex is also referred to as a salmon patch, stork bite, or angel's kiss.)

Nervus simplexes are caused by dilated blood vessels underneath the skin, and will typically fade within 1–2 years, although the neck lesions may persist longer. Crying or warm baths may make the lesions temporarily more prominent.

Approximately 40–60 percent of all babies will have at least one or more of these marks, but not to worry—they are considered normal skin lesions that are of cosmetic consequence only. If they are cosmetically concerning and they persist, they can be treated with laser therapy by a dermatologist, but this should only be considered after sufficient time has been given for the lesions to disappear on their own.

LANUGO

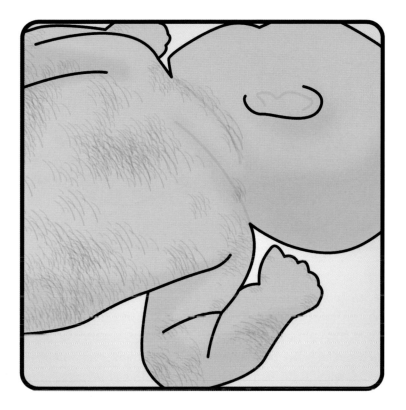

Lanugo is very thin, fine, downy hair that is sometimes found on the body of a newborn baby. Parents expecting smooth newborn skin are sometimes surprised by the amount of hair present on their baby. Typically, this hair is shed before birth, but it may be seen on any baby (although it is more common in babies who are born prematurely).

Lanugo is the first hair produced by the body, usually appearing around 4 months of gestation and found abundantly all over at 5 months of gestation. Eventually, by 3–4 months of life, all of the lanugo on the body will be replaced by vellus hair, which is thinner and less visible.

PEELING SKIN

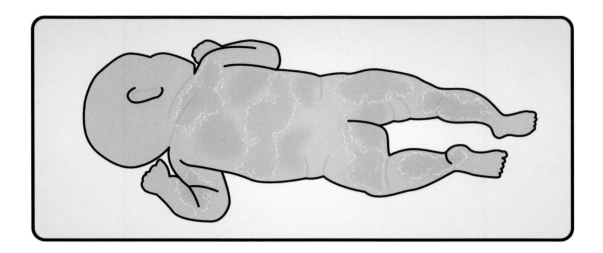

Imagine sitting in a hot tub for 9 months straight. When you finally leave the hot tub, there will understandably be a considerable amount of peeling and turnover as your skin dries up.

In essence, this is why all newborn babies have a large amount of **dry and peeling skin**. While the flaking and peeling can be cosmetically concerning, this is not a health issue. The skin can be moisturized several times a day as needed with any reputable lotion; however, even without any treatment this condition will improve within a few weeks.

Long, frequent baths can actually remove the natural oils from your baby's skin, so you may want to limit baths to every 2–3 days and keep them no longer than 5–10 minutes. Use lukewarm water and fragrance-free cleansers when possible.

Of course, if your baby absolutely adores bath time, it is reasonable to bathe them more frequently and for longer periods. In those cases, simply be more aggressive with lotions to compensate for the loss of natural oils.

MONGOLIAN SPOTS

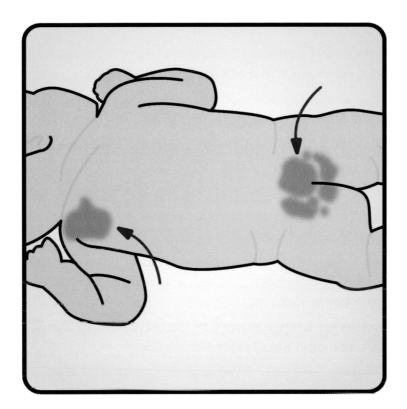

Mongolian spots are commonly seen birthmarks, typically located on the lower back, buttocks, or shoulder; less commonly, they are also seen on the arms and legs. They are usually blue in color, but can be blue-gray, blue-black, or dark brown.

These spots occur when normal pigment-making cells called melanocytes do not complete their migration to the surface of the skin and become trapped in the lower layers, leading to darkly pigmented patches.

The spots were originally named after the Mongolians, but they can be found in infants of any race. Most will disappear by 5 years of age; some can persist until puberty. Other than the cosmetic issues these spots present, there are no health concerns. Some children who have a plethora of Mongolian spots may benefit by a doctor's letter for caretakers (to alleviate any unfounded concerns of abuse, as the spots may be mistaken for bruises).

TAKE-HOME POINTS

★ Cradle cap (seborrheic dermatitis) is a cosmetic issue that will resolve on its own with time, but which can be controlled with an anti-dandruff shampoo and gentle brushing.

★ Eczema is a generalized sensitivity of the skin that typically improves with time. Flare-ups can be controlled with lotion and steroid creams.

★ Erythema toxicum is a very common rash that disappears on its own in 1–2 weeks.

★ Sebaceous gland hyperplasia is a collection of yellowish-white dots on the nose caused by maternal hormones, which will resolve on its own without treatment.

★ Milia are small bumps filled with a minute amount of trapped skin that will resolve on their own without treatment.

★ Neonatal acne, now called neonatal cephalic pustulosis, peaks at about 1 month of age and can last several months. The rash will resolve with time on its own, but can benefit from a mild steroid cream.

★ Nevus simplexes are pink-red patches on the skin caused by dilated blood vessels underneath the skin and typically fade within 1–2 years.

★ Lanugo is very thin, downy hair found on a newborn's body that will be shed by 3–4 months of life.

★ Peeling skin is a normal process that occurs after birth and can be treated with lotion and by limiting baths to every 2–3 days for the first few weeks of life.

★ Mongolian spots are benign birthmarks, typically located on the lower back, buttocks, or shoulder.

What to Know Before Having Your Baby

Chapter 3

HEAD

AS YOU look lovingly into your newborn's eyes, your gaze may fall uncomfortably upon some green mucus or a red spot on their eye. Or, as you're cradling your baby's head in the palm of your hand, you may get freaked out by an unusual bump or ridge of the skull. At times, as your baby is sleeping peacefully, you may hear strange, Darth Vader-like noises emanating from their nose and mouth.

And, understandably, you are concerned.

When a baby is born, their anatomy is small and they are still in the process of adjusting to the world. As a result, many of their facial drainage pipes and sinuses get clogged up, creating discharge and strange noises. Additionally, during the first few years of life, the body matures and undergoes a host of anatomical changes, such as the fusion of the skull's many bones.

In other words, it's only a matter of time. As your baby's vision improves, their eyes will be better aligned; as their ear canal grows, the smell will improve; and as their hormones normalize, their hair will re-grow. Before you know it, the boogers will be gone, the breathing will sound normal, and your baby will be smiling right back into your loving eyes.

HAIR LOSS

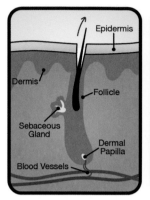

Telogen (Resting) Phase:
Dead Hair Falling Out

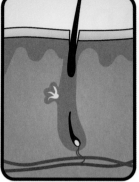

Catagen ▶ Anagen Phase:
New Hair Formation

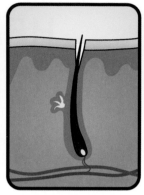

Anagen (Active Growth)
Phase: Hair Growth

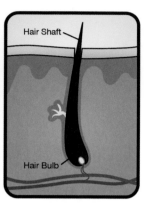

Normal Follicle

Hair growth occurs in three phases:

1. **Anagen phase**, also known as the active growth phase

2. **Catagen phase**, also known as the transition phase

3. **Telogen phase**, also known as the resting phase

At any given time, about 85 percent of your hair is in the active growth phase, which is when your hairs have the deepest roots and are actively growing. The other 15 percent of your hair will have moved through the transition phase into the resting phase, which is when your hairs have the shallowest roots, are no longer growing and easily fall out of your scalp.

What does this have to do with your baby? Well, newborn babies go through hormonal fluctuations soon after birth (as do their moms!), which leads to a one-time transition of a large percentage of their hairs into the resting phase. This causes a temporary but noticeable loss of hair during the first 6 months of life, particularly in areas where babies like to rub their heads against the mattress, which often gives them a unique posterior bald stripe for a few months.

As hormones recalibrate and normalize, your baby's hair will transition into the typical 85/15 percent growth pattern and their temporary baldness will subside. Moms will often notice the same change in their own hair growth pattern, as their hormones will go through a similar phenomenon.

What to Know Before Having Your Baby

FONTANELLE AND SKULL SUTURES

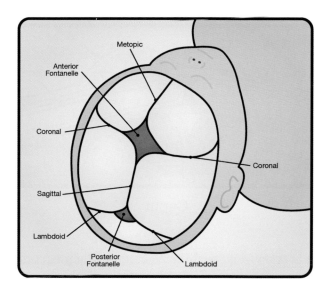

Although the skull appears to be one bone, it is actually made up of a conglomerate of five smaller bones fused together: two frontal bones, two parietal bones, and one occipital bone. These smaller bones cover the brain and are held tightly together by thick fibrous material called sutures.

Sutures are what allow the bones to move during the birthing process, allowing the head to make it out safely. They are also the primary expansion points as the head grows during the first few years of life. There are four main sutures, which extend from either front to back or side to side: the **metopic** suture, the **coronal** suture, the **sagittal** suture, and the **lambdoid** suture.

When your baby is born, you will be able to feel ridges and bumps where their skull bones overlap each other. This is normal, and should smooth out nicely by 18–24 months of age.

The spaces between the bones of an infant's skull where the sutures intersect are called **fontanelles**, of which there are two. The anterior fontanelle, also called the soft spot, occurs at the junction where the two frontal and two parietal bones meet, located near the front of the head. The anterior fontanelle remains soft until about 18–24 months of age. The soft spot is covered by thick, tough tissue that protects the brain tissue underneath, so you do not need to worry about hurting it. If you sometimes notice slight pulsations of the soft spot, not to fear; this is normal.

The posterior fontanelle, by contrast, occurs at the junction of the two parietal bones and the occipital bone, and is located near the rear of the head. Most parents will not notice the posterior fontanelle, as it is much smaller than the anterior fontanelle and will close within the first several months of life.

CAPUT SUCCEDANEUM

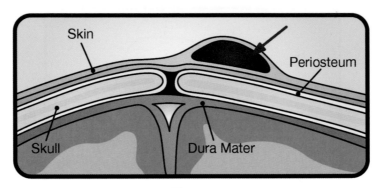

Caput

A **caput succedaneum** is a common birth complication which occurs when the baby's head pushes against the cervix/pelvis of the mother, or when the cervix applies pressure around the scalp leading to a swelling of the head. (Vacuum extraction can also lead to the formation of a caput succedaneum.)

This injury causes blood and serum to collect in the area of the scalp above the outer covering of the bone (called the periosteum), which can therefore cross the midline of the skull. They can appear quite large, at times giving the baby a temporary cone-head shape. Caput succedaneums are not harmful and resolve very quickly—usually within a few days—with the scalp fully returning to its original intended shape.

CEPHALOHEMATOMA

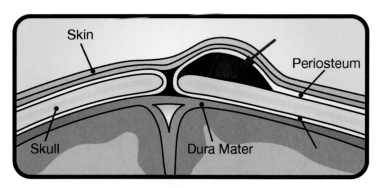

Cephalohematoma

A **cephalohematoma** is a common complication of birth, which occurs when the blood vessels between the skull bone and the outer covering of the bone (called the periosteum) rupture. This leads to a collection of blood, which appears as a soft boggy mass at the top of the head. Unlike a caput succedaneum, cephalohematoma occur *below* the periosteum, and thus follow the shape of the bone. They therefore do not cross the midline of the skull.

For the most part, cephalohematomas are benign and will resolve with time over the course of several weeks. Initially, as the swelling goes down, the outer edges of the mass may harden up as the blood calcifies. This can leave the mass with a soft, mushy center, and it may appear that there is a fracture or some other kind of injury in the middle. However, this is normal and will heal appropriately with time.

Occasionally, a cephalohematoma will lead to the destruction of a large number of red blood cells. As the red blood cells die, they will become the waste product **bilirubin**, which can in turn increase the risk of jaundice (see page 9). Should this occur, phototherapy and close monitoring of the jaundice may be necessary.

FLAT HEAD

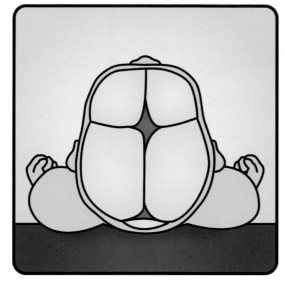
Normal Skull Shape

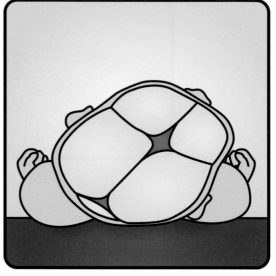
Positional Flattening - Distorted Skull Shape

Since it has become common for babies to sleep on their backs, many are developing **flat spots** on the backs of their heads. While not medically concerning, who wants their baby to have a flat head?

From the time your child is born, try to alternate the side of the head that is receiving pressure during sleep, feeding, play, and travel. For example, alternate which arm you use to hold your baby during feedings. Use a rolled up rag or small towel (tightly wound up so that it cannot suffocate the child) to control the orientation of your baby's head in their car seat. If your baby likes to gaze at a certain window, door, or fan while in bed, turn the bed around so that they must turn their head in the other direction.

Flat heads will almost always round out nicely by 3 years of age without any intervention. And yet, a lucrative industry selling "molding helmets" has sprung up, catering to nervous parents who desire a beautiful round head for their baby. In some severe cases, a helmet *may* be cosmetically beneficial; however, in most children their heads will look very nice without intervention, especially after the hair has grown out. A pediatrician can help determine when a helmet consultation may be desirable.

CRANIOSYNOSTOSIS

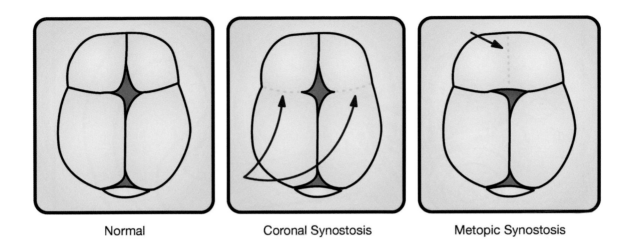

Normal   Coronal Synostosis   Metopic Synostosis

Craniosynostosis happens when one or more skull sutures close prematurely, leading to a misshapen skull. If only one suture is affected, the problem is only cosmetic; however, if two sutures are affected, it can constrict the space needed for the brain's growth leading to developmental issues and brain damage.

Luckily, craniosynostosis is quite uncommon and most cases of a misshapen skull are due to positional flattening from laying the baby on their back. By measuring the head circumference periodically and examining the skull, a pediatrician can determine whether further testing or intervention is necessary.

SMELLY EARS

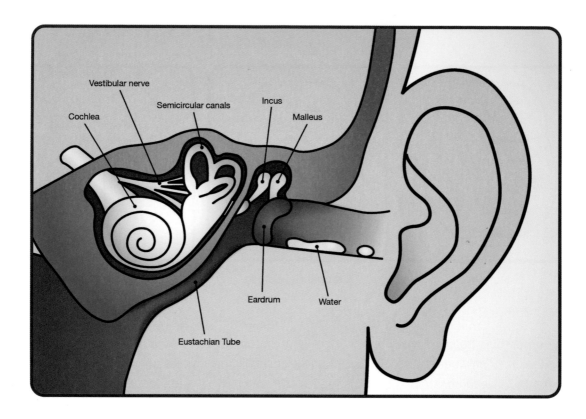

Babies in general smell very nice all over, except for a few notable places. Some of these are obvious; others are not. The ears, for example, often emit a mild to moderate foul odor as a result of **stagnant water in the outer ear canal**.

When you bathe your baby, water will inevitably get inside the canal. Because of the narrow width of the canal, this water will not quickly evaporate. As a result, the ears will often have a "wet rag" smell coming from the canals. If you dig your fingers deep into your own canals, you will find the same smell coming from your own ears too!

While this may not smell nice, there is no cause for concern, and there is no need to treat this condition. Parents *will* sometimes aggressively clean the ears after bath time. While it is perfectly safe to dry and clean the outermost area of the ear canal, it is better not to put a cotton applicator or other cleaning devices into the canal. This will only push earwax deep into the canal, possibly leading to a blockage. Aggressive cleaning can also irritate or break the skin, possibly precipitating a skin infection.

Also, bear in mind that some water entering the ear canal is desirable as it will help the wax to migrate outward, keeping the ear clean.

EARWAX

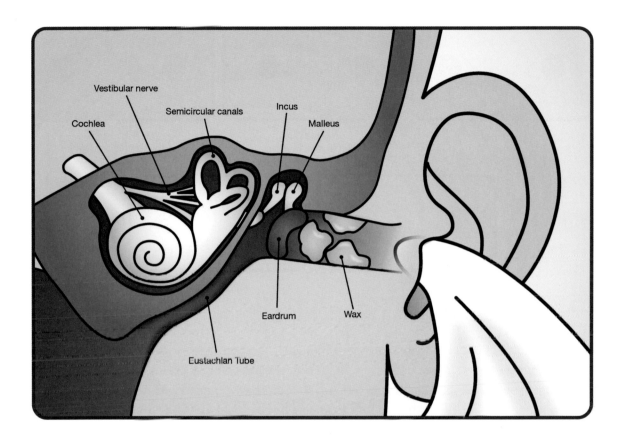

For all the scorn that **earwax** receives, it actually has many important functions. Earwax helps protect the ear canal by providing a waterproof lining, trapping dirt and other particles, in addition to possessing antibacterial properties which reduces the risk of infections.

Your body is purposefully and perpetually making earwax, which will naturally work its way out of the ear canal over time. Water getting in the ear canal during bathing time will help facilitate this natural migration; as such, getting some water in the ears is safe, and even desirable.

When earwax is present at the visible part of the ear canal, simply take a wet washcloth and carefully clean the area. As mentioned previously, cleaning the ear with a cotton applicator or other cleaning device can lead to blockages and infections.

Most kids make just the right amount of earwax. A small percentage of children will overproduce earwax and may need some medical assistance in preventing the ear canal from getting blocked.

CROSS-EYED

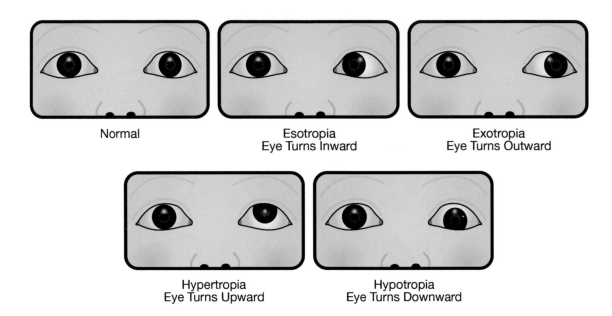

Normal

Esotropia
Eye Turns Inward

Exotropia
Eye Turns Outward

Hypertropia
Eye Turns Upward

Hypotropia
Eye Turns Downward

Parents are often concerned when they see that their newborn's eyes aren't tracking together as well as they expect. When babies are first born, their vision is extremely poor and they can only focus on objects 8–12 inches from their face. Additionally, the muscles that move their eyes are immature. As a result, their eyes will often wander and *appear* to be misaligned, especially during the first 4 months of life. As their vision improves, so will the alignment of their eyes, and by 4 months of age the eyes should track together.

If your child's eyes appear misaligned past 4 months of life, a visit to the pediatrician is warranted. Any persistent misalignment of the eyes past 4 months of age can be a sign of a condition called **strabismus** and may need to be evaluated by a pediatric ophthalmologist.

What to Know Before Having Your Baby

PSEUDOSTRABISMUS

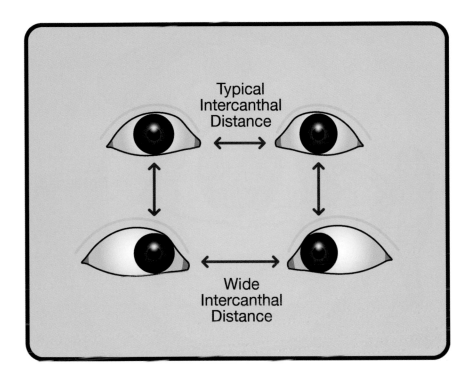

True **strabismus** is a condition in which the eyes are not aligned correctly, and which is indicative of a medical issue that must be evaluated by a pediatric ophthalmologist. **Pseudostrabismus**, on the other hand, is not a true medical issue and does not need to be treated.

In pseudostrabismus, an optical illusion makes the eyes appear to be misaligned or cross-eyed, even though the eyes are actually centered appropriately. The most common cause is when the area of the skin between the eyes, known as the **intercanthal distance**, is wider than the average baby's, which gives the illusion that the pupils are closer together than they actually are.

Pseudostrabismus can be seen in any race, but it is most common in Native Americans and East Asians. As facial features mature, the widened nasal bridge will become narrower and the pseudostrabismus will become less noticeable.

CRUSTY EYES AND BLOCKED TEAR DUCTS

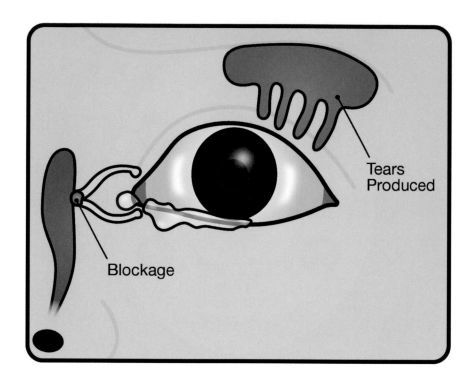

Tears Produced

Blockage

To keep your eyes moist, your body continually makes a small amount of tears, which then drain down the tear ducts into your nose. In essence, tear ducts are the drainage pipes for your eyes.

Because babies are small, they have tiny tear ducts. As such, the ducts become blocked quite easily with debris and mucus. During the first year of life, it is quite common for babies to wake up with yellow goop crusted around their eye(s). Some babies will also appear to tear from one or both eyes even when they are not crying. As babies get physically larger, so will their tear ducts and eventually the problem should go away on its own by 12 months of age—if not sooner.

However, if in addition to yellow goop there is also redness and/or swelling of the skin around the eye, an infection may be present. This is not very common, but if seen, it should be evaluated by a pediatrician as soon as possible.

To treat a blocked tear duct, gently massage the area between the affected eye and nose for several minutes, 3–4 times a day. Applying a warm towel while you massage may also help, although this is not necessary.

If the blocked tear duct(s) is still present at 1 year of life, a visit to the pediatric ophthalmologist may be warranted. But, in the vast majority of children, the problem will improve on its own with no intervention.

What to Know Before Having Your Baby

SUBCONJUNCTIVAL HEMORRHAGE

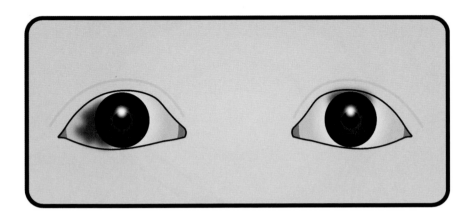

Subconjunctival hemorrhages appear as bloody marks on the white part of the eyeball. They are quite common in newborns and occur when small vessels in the eye break during the pressure of delivery. The red area can be quite large at times, covering almost the entire side of the eyeball—but like a small bruise, it will get better on its own over the course of several days. At times, some color changes (similar to that of a bruise healing) may be noted.

Subconjunctival hemorrhages do not affect vision and are not painful. Sometimes, other facial signs of delivery pressure will also be present, such as a bruise on the face or a patch of tiny purple-red dots covering the forehead. These are also not cause for concern.

NASAL CONGESTION

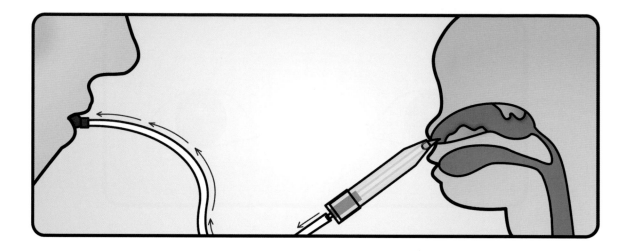

During the first 2–3 months of life, most newborn babies will have some **nasal mucus** that can cause sneezing and noisy breathing. They are not allergic to anything—they are simply adjusting to all of the particles in the air, which can irritate the nasal passages. Often they will sound like Darth Vader when they are breathing! Remember that babies are small; as such, their nasal passages are tiny. Consequently, even small amounts of mucus can lead to noisy breathing.

To alleviate this, use a nasal suction device (along with nasal saline from the pharmacy) to clean the nasal passages. Leave 1–2 drops of nasal saline on each side of the nose for 15–30 seconds, and then suction the nose. Note, however, that some of the mucus may be too far back to reach with suctioning. A cool mist vaporizer in your baby's room may also help, as can elevating the head of the bed. Although nothing may appear to work great, take solace in the fact that this will improve as the baby gets physically larger and their nasal passages widen.

HICCUPS

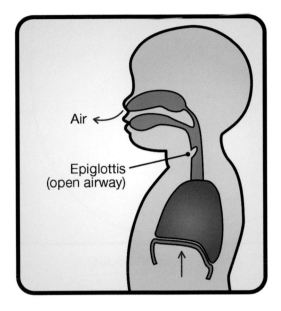 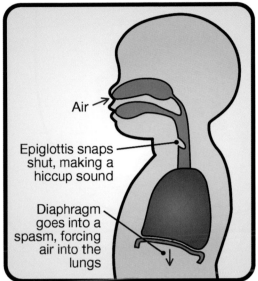

Hiccups are caused by an involuntary contraction of the diaphragm followed by a closure of the vocal cords, leading to the classic "hic" sound. Hiccups can be caused by a number of things, but the most common causes for infants include crying, swallowing air, reflux, and eating too quickly.

Hiccups are not dangerous and generally bother the parents more than the baby. They will resolve with time and no treatment is necessary. To reduce the frequency of hiccups, parents can burp their baby more frequently, use a slower flow nipple, or try different positions when feeding. Regardless of what methods are employed, parents should still expect regular episodes of hiccups that will become less frequent with maturity.

EPSTEIN'S PEARLS AND BOHN'S NODULES

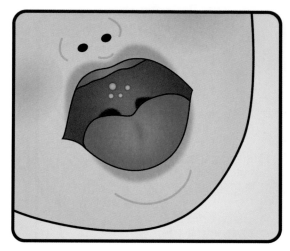

Epstein's Pearls

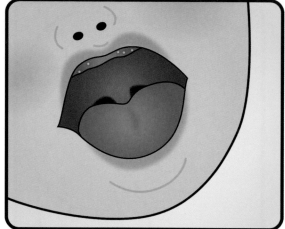

Bohn's Nodules

Epstein's pearls and **Bohn's nodules** occur when skin cells become trapped, and appear as tiny white bumps inside the mouth. Epstein's pearls occur at the roof of the mouth in the midline area, whereas Bohn's nodules occur along the gums.

Bohn's nodules are often confused as teeth because of their location on the gums. However, when rubbed a Bohn's nodule is softer than the enamel of a tooth, and has a characteristic circular appearance.

Neither Epstein's pearls nor Bohn's nodules are cause for concern, and both will resolve in a few weeks on their own.

TONGUE-TIE

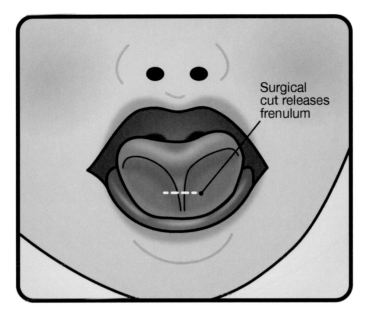

Surgical cut releases frenulum

Lingual Frenulum

Anywhere from 1–10 percent of babies are born with **tongue-tie**, which is where the base or tip of the tongue is persistently attached to the bottom of the mouth. Tongue-tie can restrict both side-to-side tongue movement and the ability to protrude the tongue out of the mouth. If severe, it can interfere with feeding (particularly breastfeeding) and lead to pronunciation issues when the child begins talking.

Because there are not a lot of well-done studies on tongue-tie, experts have a wide range of opinions as to how concerning tongue-tie is and how aggressively it should be treated. Certainly, if there are any feeding issues stemming from a tongue-tie issue, then an evaluation by an experienced lactation consultant, pediatric dentist, or otolaryngologist (ENT surgeon) should be completed as soon as possible.

However, if a child is feeding well and gaining good weight, there is little urgency to the issue. Many experts believe that mild cases of tongue-tie will resolve with time as the tongue naturally stretches out and becomes more mobile.

While a severe tongue-tie can hamper pronunciation, especially with lingual sounds such as the letter "t" and "n", it will not delay speech or prevent the child from making sounds.

Tongue-tie can be surgically corrected with a simple procedure, usually done in the doctor's office without the need for general anesthesia; however, severe cases may need to be taken to the operating room. The timing and need for surgery should be determined on a case-by-case basis.

THRUSH

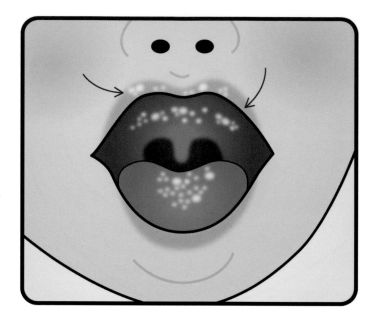

It is common and even normal for the tongue of a newborn baby to be white at times, either from breast milk or formula coating the tongue or from changes in the papillae (which are the fingerlike projections that make up the surface of the tongue). However, if the white coating on the tongue is markedly thick and begins to spread to the cheeks, roof of the mouth, or the lips, it is likely caused by an infection called **thrush**.

Oral thrush is caused by a common fungus called **Candida**, which often resides harmlessly in our mouth and on our skin without causing any problems. However, when the immune system is weak (such as in a newborn baby), Candida can grow unchecked and can organize into plaques which quickly overtake our mouth and skin. In babies, this typically happens in the mouth and/or diaper area—leading to an angry-looking red diaper rash.

Thrush is easily treated with an antifungal medication called Nystatin which, because it is not readily absorbed by the intestinal tract, is very safe to use. A typical course will be to apply the Nystatin to the white plaques four times a day for 2 weeks. Breastfeeding mothers may also want to treat their nipples. To prevent a recurrence, all bottles and pacifiers should be thoroughly washed.

As the baby's immune system matures and the body becomes fully colonized with healthy bacteria, the risk of thrush (and Candida diaper rashes) will decrease.

TEETHING AND CLEANING

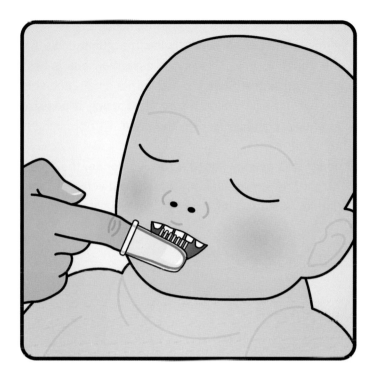

Although **teething** typically starts between 4–6 months of age, there is a lot of variability as to when teeth erupt, with some children being born with teeth and others not having their first tooth until after their first birthday. Regardless of when teething starts, virtually all babies will eventually get all 20 of their primary teeth by 2–3 years of age.

If children are born with teeth, it is a good idea to see a pediatric dentist, as they may need to be removed. This does not occur very frequently; more often than not, any "teeth" seen at birth may actually be Bohn's nodules (see page 40). Some parents worry about late teethers; they should consider this a small blessing, as they can start brushing teeth later in life!

All babies will drool, especially as their salivary glands grow, but this is not necessarily a sign that teeth are about to come in. As babies get more nimble, they will begin to explore the world by sticking everything they can grab into their mouths. This, too, is not a specific sign that teeth are about to come in. Drooling and chewing on things may increase some as teeth come in, but babies will drool and chew on things in general, just by nature of being a baby!

Some babies will have a hard time with teething and become quite irritable as the teeth cut through their gums. However, most babies take teething in stride with just a bit of fussiness. In general, topical numbing gels can cause a variety of side effects—some quite serious—so it is best to avoid using them. The best remedies are to allow babies to chew on refrigerated teething rings (do *not* freeze them, or you risk freezer burns) and to take a pain reliever such as acetaminophen (or ibuprofen, if older than 6 months) as needed.

Before teething begins, parents can simply wipe the gums down with a wet washcloth twice a day to keep the gums healthy. This is not essential, but *is* helpful. As teeth erupt, parents should begin brushing the teeth twice a day with a small, rice-sized amount of fluoride toothpaste. After three years of age, children can start using a pea-size amount of fluoride toothpaste, but parents should continue to help the child with brushing their teeth until they can spit out well on their own.

As a last note: although it is optimal not to swallow fluoride, the American Dental Association announced in 2014 that the benefits of early fluoride outweigh the small risk of swallowing toothpaste (topical fluoride, when swallowed, can potentially cause white stains on future permanent teeth).

What to Know Before Having Your Baby

TEETH STAINS

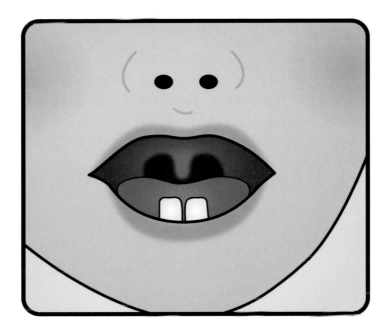

Teeth can **stain** for any number of reasons, and baby (primary) teeth are no exception. Most stains are generally a cosmetic issue only, and not an actual medical issue. However, babies and toddlers can develop cavities, which *will* require treatment. The risk of this happening is based on a mixture of diet, genetics, and dental hygiene habits.

Stains can be an array of colors, including white, gray, green, orange, brown, yellow, and black. Some of the primary causes of stains are listed below:

- **Plaques:** If teeth are not brushed properly, plaques of various colors will form on the teeth. These can be cleared by brushing the teeth or, for hardier plaques, with proper tools at the dentist's office.

- **Cavities:** If plaques are not adequately removed, cavities can form which appear as dark brown/black pits or crevices in the enamel of the teeth.

- **Medications:** Certain medications are known to stain teeth, such as vitamins or certain types of antibiotics.

- **Injury**: Trauma to baby teeth can cause a brown or gray discoloration, which is not superficial and cannot be brushed off.

- **Excess Fluoride**: Too much fluoride in the diet or from too much toothpaste ingestion can lead to faint white markings or streaks on the teeth.

- **Illness**: Certain types of illnesses unrelated to teeth can cause staining of the teeth.

When stains appear on baby teeth, parents should attempt to remove the stains by brushing thoroughly with a rice-grain sized dab of toothpaste. If the stains cannot be removed after several tooth brushing sessions, it is generally a good idea to visit a pediatric dentist to find out if anything further needs to be done.

What to Know Before Having Your Baby

LYMPH NODES

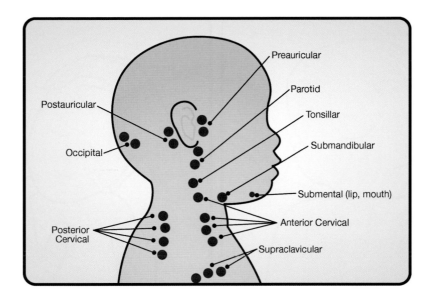

Lymph nodes are essentially the battle stations for your immune system. They are located throughout your body from head to toe and feel like soft rubber balls under the skin. In certain areas, you can easily feel them, such as under the armpits, beneath the jawbone, behind the ears, at the back of the head, and in your groin area. (The lymph nodes at the back of the head are a common source of anxiety for parents; a quick exam by their pediatrician can help put their mind at ease.)

Blood cells called **lymphocytes** are created in our bone marrow and thymus, before migrating to hang out in our lymph nodes. As germs are detected in our body, they are routed to our lymph nodes, where lymphocytes create large amounts of antibodies, which are then sent out to the rest of our body to label germs so that they will be extinguished. This process causes the lymph nodes near the infection to swell.

Often, the immune system does such a good job getting rid of the germ that these swollen lymph nodes are the only sign of an infection. They will return to normal size over the course of several weeks or months after the germs have been properly defeated.

However, from time to time it is possible for the lymph nodes themselves to become infected, in which case they will become quite red, warm, and tender to the touch. Additionally, if several lymph nodes become swollen all at once, it can be a sign of certain illnesses. Both of these scenarios should be brought to the attention of the pediatrician.

In general, lymph nodes swelling up are a sign that you are healthy and your immune system is working properly!

TORTICOLLIS

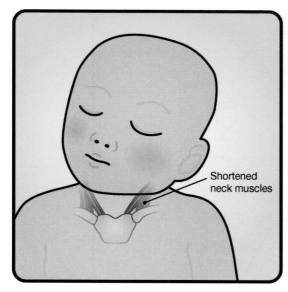
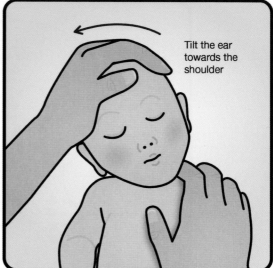

Shortened neck muscles

Tilt the ear towards the shoulder

Torticollis literally means "twisted neck" in Latin. Babies with torticollis will appear to have a head that is tilted to one side, and will prefer to lie on the same side of their head every night. Torticollis can happen by itself, or you may see it paired up with a flat head (see page 30) or possibly with a hip issue called developmental dyplasia of the hips (see page 85).

The main muscle that is involved is called the sternocleidomastoid muscle, which runs from the back of the ears to the collarbone. At times, parents may notice a bump or knot on the muscle, which is a normal finding with torticollis and is not a cause for alarm.

Even without therapy, most torticollis will improve with time as kids become more mobile and active and begin using their neck muscles more and more. However, stretching exercises can help the torticollis to improve more quickly. While laying the baby on a firm surface, parents can tilt the head toward the shoulder and apply steady pressure with their hand for one minute to the right and one minute to the left. Do this with each diaper change (or 6–8 times a day).

Torticollis can appear at birth, or as late as 3 months of life. It is likely caused by the position the baby was lying in within the womb, but there may be other contributing factors. In severe cases, physical therapy or rarely surgery may be necessary. Most cases will improve quickly, and before parents even realize it, the neck will straighten out and move appropriately.

TAKE-HOME POINTS

★ Hair loss triggered by hormonal fluctuations is common in the first 6 months of life, but it is temporary and the hair will grow back.

★ Ridges and bumps called sutures and soft spots called fontanelles are normal and should smooth out nicely by 18–24 months of age.

★ A caput succedaneum is a common complication of birth, which results from an injury to the scalp leading to a collection of blood and serum. These are not harmful and will usually resolve within a few days.

★ A cephalohematoma is a common complication of birth, which results from a rupture of the blood vessels between the skull bone and the outer covering of the bone (called the periosteum). These are not harmful and will usually resolve within a few weeks.

★ Many babies will get some position-induced flattening of the skull from lying on their backs. Most flat heads will round out nicely on their own by three years of age.

★ Smelly ears result from water getting trapped within the ear canal. In general, it is best to only clean the outside of the ear canal.

★ Earwax has helpful properties and only needs to be removed if the canal is completely blocked. Luckily, most children's ears are self-cleaning and only the outside of the ear canal needs to be cleaned.

★ Babies are born with poor vision and immature eye muscles. As such, they will often appear to be cross-eyed. This should resolve on its own by 4 months of age.

★ Pseudostrabismus may be appreciated when there is a wide intercanthal distance between the eyes creating an optical illusion of the baby appearing cross-eyed. This is not a medical issue, and there is no cause for concern.

★ Blocked tear ducts occur when the natural drainage pipe of the eyes become clogged, leading to yellow goop buildup in the eyes. In most children, this will resolve by 12 months of age.

- ★ Subconjunctival hemorrhages are burst blood vessels of the eye caused by the pressure of the delivery process. They are not harmful or painful and will resolve quickly on their own.

- ★ Nasal congestion in newborns occurs from small amounts of mucus clogging up their small nasal passages. As their body grows the nasal passages will get larger and the congestion will improve on its own.

- ★ Hiccups occur quite frequently in newborns but are not dangerous and are not a sign of any health issues. As babies mature, the frequency of hiccups will decrease.

- ★ Epstein's pearls and Bohn's nodules are trapped skin cells that appear as white dots on the roof of the mouth and gums, respectively. They are benign and will go away on their own.

- ★ Any tongue-ties leading to feeding or speech issues should be treated. However, if a child is feeding well and gaining good weight, there is low urgency to the issue.

- ★ Oral thrush is a common fungal infection of the mouth that appears as a white plaque, and is easily treated with an antifungal medication called Nystatin.

- ★ There is a lot of variability when teething begins, and any delay should not worry parents, as virtually all children will eventually get all of their primary teeth.

- ★ In 2014, the American Dental Association recommended using a rice grain-sized amount of fluoride toothpaste twice a day for brushing a baby's teeth.

- ★ Teeth stains can occur for any number of reasons and most are not concerning. If the stains cannot be removed after several tooth-brushing sessions, a pediatric dentist should be seen.

- ★ Lymph nodes are located throughout your body and feel like soft rubber balls underneath your skin. Lymph nodes are a normal part of your body and are an important part of your immune system.

- ★ A baby with torticollis will appear to have their head tilted to one side. In severe cases, physical therapy or (rarely) surgery may be necessary; however, most cases will improve on their own in due time.

What to Know Before Having Your Baby

Chapter 4

TORSO

AS YOUR baby begins to eat and put on some weight, you will notice your baby sporting a quickly growing belly. Before they round out nicely, you may notice a strange notch in the center of their chest, or perhaps your attention will be drawn to the swollen nipples they were born with. And of course, you will notice the daily changes their umbilical cord undergoes as it dries up, shrivels up, and falls off. None of these are cause for alarm, but as your baby grows and matures, it helps to have an understanding of their changing body.

ENLARGED BREASTS

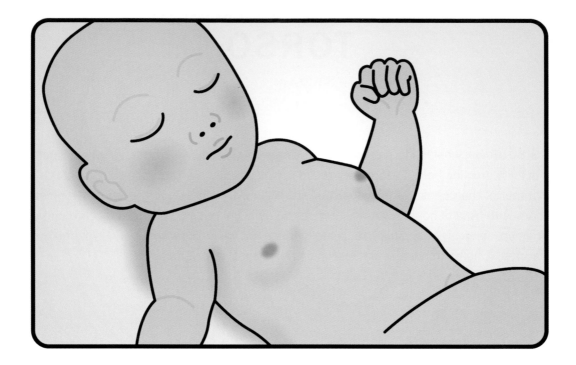

The same hormones which cause a new mom to have enlarged breasts can cross over the placenta and induce **swelling of the breasts in infants** (both male and female). This is very common, and is temporary; some babies will even have small amounts of actual milk secrete from their breasts.

Typically after a few weeks (but sometimes longer), the breasts will begin to shrink as the exposure to the hormones decreases. Even after the swelling has reduced, parents may notice a small remnant of breast tissue left over. This is also normal, and not a cause for concern.

Some parents may try to manipulate the breasts to express the milk in hopes of decreasing the swelling faster. This can lead to irritation of the breast tissue and occasionally trigger an infection. It is best to leave the breasts alone and allow them to shrink naturally with time.

If at any point any redness or rapid swelling is noted, especially if the breasts appear to be tender and painful to touch, a visit to the pediatrician is warranted.

NORMAL MURMURS

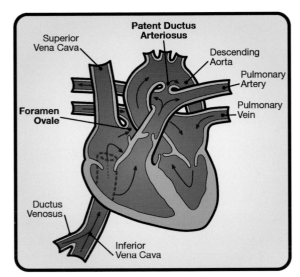

Fetal Heart Before Birth

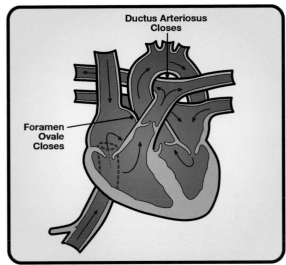

Newborn Heart After Birth

Just like you can hear water running through pipes or wind flowing through a duct, it is common to hear blood moving through the heart. A **heart murmur** is an extra sound heard during the regular heartbeat cycle. It is typically a whooshing sound, created by some kind of turbulence in your blood flow. Although it can be representative of heart disease, the vast majority of heart murmurs are normal sounds, and are not indicative of any problem or defect.

To understand the common defects that may affect a heart, imagine the heart muscle as four rooms, each room having two doors (or valves)—one door that leads the blood in and one door that lets the blood out. The most common concerning defects occur when one of the valves is not working properly or if one of the rooms has more than one way in or out.

When babies are first born, there is a normal transitional period for the blood flow as the body adjusts from receiving oxygen through the placenta to receiving oxygen through the lungs. This will create some turbulence, and often pediatricians will hear murmurs on the first exam that will resolve typically within 24 hours (although some innocent murmurs may last as long as several months). In fact, at some point in their life 80 percent (or more) of healthy children will have some sort of transient murmur. Innocent murmurs do not need to be treated, as there is no defect present and the heart is functioning 100 percent normally.

At times, however, a murmur may have a harsher sound to it, or there may be signs of a heart defect such as shortness of breath or a persistent bluish hue of the face and/or body. (Blue hands and feet, on the other hand, are quite common and by themselves are not a cause for concern.) If your pediatrician suspects a true heart problem, they will order some tests such as a chest x-ray, electrocardiogram (ECG), or an echocardiogram to assess the health and anatomy of the heart. More often than not, however, a newborn murmur will not cause any health issues and will resolve on its own in due course.

DISTENDED BELLY

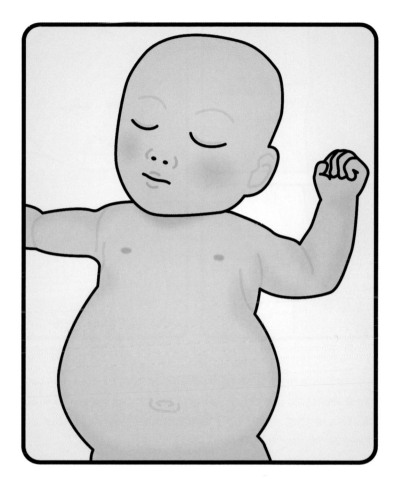

When babies are first born, their bellies will often look quite large compared to the rest of their body, giving their torso an eggplant shape. This is normal and nothing to be worried about.

Between feedings, the belly should feel soft. But when the intestines become filled with gas or stool, it is not unusual for the belly to feel taut (almost like a drum). As long as the child is eating well, passing stool, and appears comfortable, nothing needs to be done. However, if the infant is refusing to eat, has not passed a stool in several days, or is fussy and inconsolable, then contact your pediatrician for an evaluation.

DIASTASIS RECTI

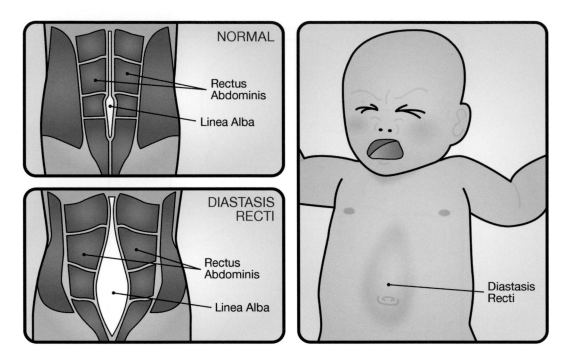

A **diastasis recti** appears as a ridge running from the bottom of the breastbone to the belly button. Essentially, a diastasis recti is a protrusion of the central area of the abdomen in between two strips of muscle tissue that make up the abdominal wall on either side. They are more noticeable when babies are crying or sitting up.

With time, most diastasis recti will improve on their own as the abdominal muscles begin to seal up, closing the gap. Rarely, a diastasis recti will be complicated by a hernia, which may require surgery.

UMBILICAL CORD

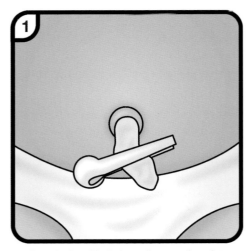

Day 1: Cord is light yellow and moist.

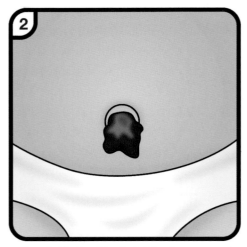

Day 4-10: Cord is dark blue/brown and is hard to the touch.

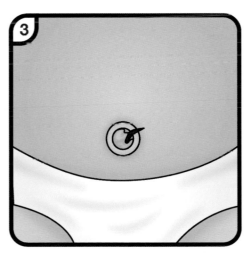

Day 10-14: Cord falls off and may leave small remnants behind. Belly button may be yellow/green and moist.

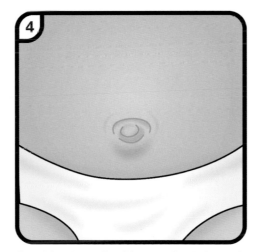

Day 14 or later: Cord is completely healed.

After clipping the umbilical cord at birth, there will be a small stump left on your baby's belly button with a small plastic clip attached to it. Most hospitals will remove the plastic clip right before discharging the baby home; if the clip has not been removed, the pediatrician can remove it in their office.

The umbilical cord will dry quickly and eventually fall off on its own, typically in 1–2 weeks, but sometimes it can take as long as 4 weeks. Older recommendations pushed aggressive cleaning of the cord, but more recent studies suggest that the only cleaning that is needed is some gentle wiping with gauze and water. Until the cord completely comes off, it is generally a good idea only to do sponge baths. Full immersion baths can start as soon as the cord falls off.

Occasionally, the umbilical cord may separate from its base and there may be a small amount of bleeding. The bleeding will typically stop on its own with no intervention, but to help it clot, parents can apply some gentle pressure to the area with a piece of gauze. If the bleeding persists longer than 15 minutes, the pediatrician should be contacted.

If at any point, the skin around the umbilical cord turns red, begins to swell, or emits a strong foul odor, a visit to the pediatrician is warranted to check for a possible infection.

UMBILICAL GRANULOMA

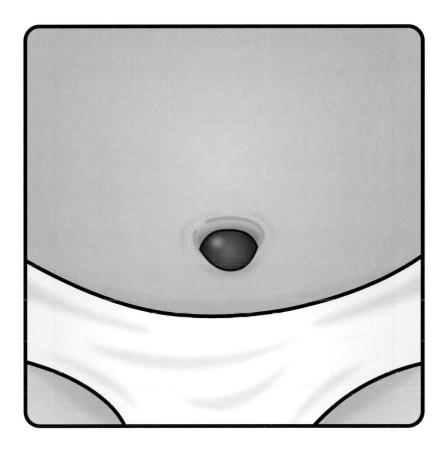

Sometimes, after the umbilical cord comes off, parents may notice a bright red bump at the base of the belly button called an **umbilical granuloma**. The granuloma may secrete a small amount of yellowish fluid, which can irritate the surrounding skin. The granuloma itself is not painful to the baby and will often heal on its own, typically within 1–2 weeks.

If the granuloma persists, the pediatrician can treat it by cauterizing it with silver nitrate or tying it off with surgical thread. Until the granuloma heals, try to keep the diaper from rubbing against it and gently clean any fluid around it with some gauze and water.

If at any point the skin around the umbilical cord turns red, begins to swell, or emits a strong foul odor, a visit to the pediatrician is warranted to check for a possible infection.

UMBILICAL HERNIA

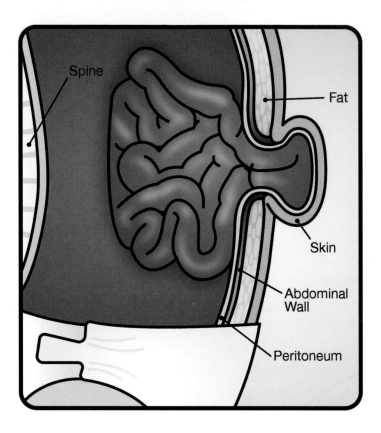

One common problem of the umbilical area is the presence of a **hernia**. When a baby is first born, the muscles where the umbilical cord inserts into the belly should seal up tightly. However, if the muscles do *not* seal appropriately, then the intestines can protrude through the opening. This is particularly noticeable when the baby cries or strains, as this increases the pressure in the abdominal area pushing the intestines outward.

Umbilical hernias are more common in babies born prematurely and in the African-American population. They are painless and do not cause any health issues in the baby.

Umbilical hernias (unlike inguinal hernias in the groin area) are not an urgent medical issue and 90 percent of cases will resolve themselves on their own by 2 years of age. If the hernia should persist past 2 years, then surgery may be necessary, albeit mostly for cosmetic reasons. It is rare to have any kind of complication from an umbilical hernia.

Some cultures will tie a coin or object on top of the umbilical area to help the hernia to improve and resolve. While this is generally not harmful—other than some mild irritation to the skin—there is also no proven benefit to this treatment.

TAKE-HOME POINTS

★ Enlarged breasts in male and female babies can occur from hormonal stimulation. If the breasts become red or tender, they should be examined; otherwise, the swelling should resolve with time.

★ Most early heart murmurs are normal and are not representative of a heart defect. However, if a baby is also short of breath or has a bluish hue of the face and/or body, a pediatrician should be seen immediately.

★ Most babies will have large, distended bellies that can even feel taut like a drum. As long as the child is eating well, passing stool, and appears comfortable, then nothing needs to be done.

★ The xiphoid process is the cartilage extension of the breastbone (sternum) and is a normal part of the anatomy.

★ A diastasis recti appears as a ridge running from the bottom of the breastbone to the belly button. Most diastasis recti will improve on their own as the abdominal muscles begin to seal up and close the gap.

★ Umbilical cords will typically dry up and fall off on their own in 1–2 weeks, but can sometimes take as long as 4 weeks. Despite older recommendations, they do not need to be cleaned (other than with gauze and water).

★ After the umbilical cord comes off, there may be an umbilical granuloma at the base of the belly button. Most will heal on their own, but when necessary can be treated with silver nitrate or by tying it off with surgical thread.

★ Umbilical hernias occur when the muscles around the belly button do not seal together tightly, appearing as a protrusion of the belly button itself. The majority of these will resolve on their own by 2 years of age.

Chapter 5

DIAPER AREA

THE AREA of the body that prompts the most questions from parents is the diaper area. Early on, parents are often concerned about the stool's frequency, color, smell, and texture. Many will track every poop and pee that their baby creates, and will often create accompanying graphs!

This diligence is impressive; however, usually by the third baby the charts and graphs will be gone, replaced by a Zen sense of calm and wisdom.

For the most part, if your baby has peed and pooped in the hospital, there is little to be worried about, as this proves all of the piping is working appropriately. At times, babies will battle a bit of gas, a bout of constipation, and the occasional diaper rash. Luckily, there are some helpful tricks (mixed with a dash of grandma's wisdom) that can help sort things out quickly.

So feel free to use those iPhone apps to monitor the changes in your baby's poo, but rest assured that if they are gaining weight and growing, there is little to be worried about.

What to Know Before Having Your Baby

HYMENAL SKIN TAG

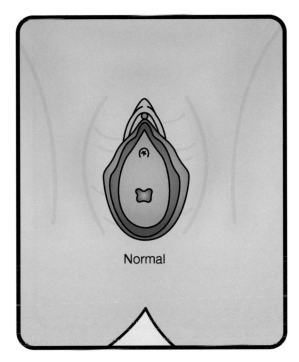

Normal

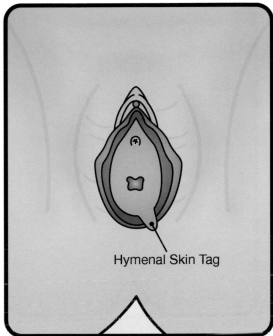

Hymenal Skin Tag

Hymenal skin tags are seen in roughly 3–13 percent of healthy female newborns. Parents may notice a small, finger-shaped piece of moist skin protruding from the vaginal area. Hymenal skin tags can be seen at either the superior (closer to the belly button) or inferior (closer to the anus) aspect of the vagina, but they are more commonly located at the inferior aspect.

Although hymenal skin tags are typically noticed right after birth, the external hymenal ridge may slowly extend outward over time and a tag may be noticed for the first time at several days or weeks of life.

Hymenal skin tags are benign and will not cause any medical issues. They do not need to be treated or removed; as the child grows, the tag will become less apparent with time.

LABIAL ADHESIONS

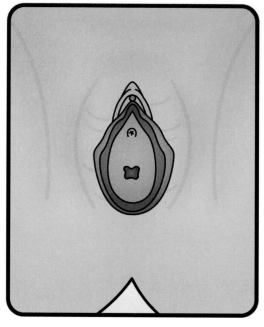
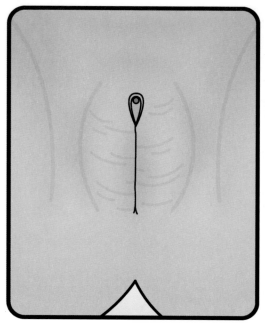

Normal Labia   Labial Adhesion

Labial adhesions are present in approximately 3 percent of prepubertal females, typically presenting between 3 months to 3 years of life. Labial adhesions present as a fusion of the skin at the opening of the vagina, appearing as if superglue is holding the two sides together. Labial adhesions are generally benign, and 80 percent of cases will resolve within 1 year with little or no intervention.

In rare cases, labial adhesions may cause a blockage of the flow of urine, which can lead to toilet training issues or even urinary tract infections. If the adhesions do not resolve by puberty, they may also interfere with menstruation outflow (though this is very uncommon).

The majority of cases will resolve on their own as the child matures and begins to secrete their own estrogen, which will help the skin to separate. Day-to-day activities, especially as the child becomes more nimble, will also help to stretch the skin apart.

To help the process along, your pediatrician may recommend a pull-down maneuver or the application of an estrogen cream. In difficult cases, a visit to a pediatric urologist may be warranted for possible surgical intervention; however, this is typically not needed.

What to Know Before Having Your Baby

NEWBORN BLOODY SHOW

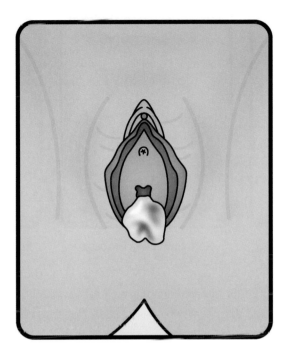

Many newborn girls present with a **whitish discharge** from their vagina, which is secondary to hormonal changes at birth. Some even have a little bloody discharge in the first few weeks of life, again as a result of withdrawal from mom's hormones. This is normal and no cause for worry; gently clean the area with a cotton ball or gauze soaked in water as needed.

CIRCUMCISION

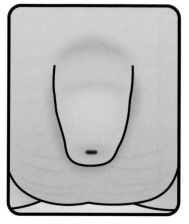
Before Circumcision

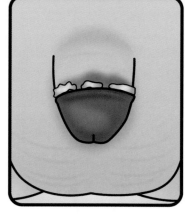
Normal Healing Process

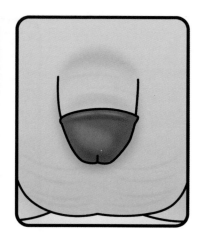
Fully-Healed Circumcision

Circumcision is an elective surgical procedure in which the skin covering the end of the penis is removed. Scientific studies have shown certain health benefits to circumcision. Additionally, parents may opt for circumcision for religious, social, or cultural reasons. Because circumcision is not essential to a child's health, parents should choose what is best for their child by weighing the benefits and risks.

Medical benefits of circumcision include:

- A markedly lower risk of acquiring HIV, the virus that causes AIDS.

- A significantly lower risk of acquiring a number of sexually transmitted infections (STIs), including genital herpes (HSV), human papilloma virus (HPV), and syphilis.

- A slightly lower risk of urinary tract infections (UTIs). A circumcised infant boy has about a 1 in 1,000 chance of developing a UTI in the first year of life; an uncircumcised infant boy has about a 1 in 100 chance of developing a UTI in the first year of life.

- A lower risk of getting cancer of the penis (however, this type of cancer is very rare in all males).

- Prevention of foreskin infections.

- Prevention of phimosis, a condition in uncircumcised males that makes foreskin retraction impossible.

- Easier genital hygiene.

If you decide to have your newborn boy circumcised, it is a good idea to do so within the first few months of life, when the procedure can be completed with local anesthesia. Typically, after 3–6 months of age, many surgeons will require general anesthesia, which carries a higher degree of risk and side effects.

For the first few days after the circumcision, you will need to regularly apply Vaseline over the circumcision. This should be done with each diaper change. After about a week, the skin should be healed well enough, and this practice can be discontinued. You will notice some yellow secretions and mild swelling surrounding the circumcised area for about one week after the circumcision.

For a circumcised child, it is important to pull the foreskin away from the head of the penis on a regular basis to prevent a bridge of scar tissue from forming at the end of the penis. You should begin doing this 2 weeks after the circumcision has healed. In an uncircumcised child, it is not recommended to pull the foreskin back until it releases on its own, which should happen naturally by 4–5 years of age.

From time to time, when the foreskin separates from the head of the penis, you may notice some white, pearl-like lumps or discharge around the head of the penis. These are shed dead skin cells and are called **smegma**. Smegma is normal and nothing to worry about and can be cleaned off with a piece of gauze and water as needed.

There are definite health benefits to circumcising your child; ultimately, however, it is a personal decision for the family to make after considering all the pros and cons.

UNDESCENDED TESTES

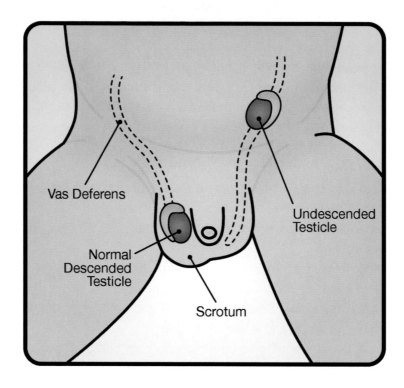

Vas Deferens

Undescended Testicle

Normal Descended Testicle

Scrotum

About 2–5 percent of full-term boys and 30 percent of premature boys will have an **undescended testicle**—meaning that one or both of the testicles cannot be felt in the scrotum. About 70 percent of these undescended testicles will come down on their own by 1 year of age, with most descending by 6 months.

Normally, the testicles will migrate from the abdominal area to the scrotum shortly before birth. In some boys, one or both testicles will stop short along the pathway and remain in the inguinal canal area (the space between your leg and your belly) or in the abdomen.

Note that testicles will often retract upward and seem hidden when the **cremasteric reflex** is triggered—which is a normal reflex in all males. A careful examination by a pediatrician can help determine if the testicle(s) are truly undescended, or if they are simply transiently displaced because of the cremasteric reflex. If the testicles can be "milked down" by the pediatrician, there is no need to be concerned.

Testicles that remain undescended need to be surgically corrected to prevent complications to the testicle, including hernias, trauma to the testicle from compression against the pelvic bone, fertility issues, and possible cancer issues in the future.

HYDROCELE

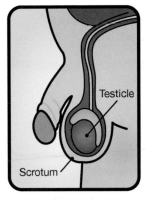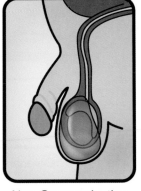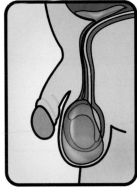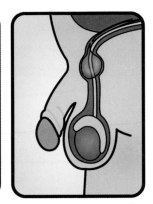

| Normal | Non-Communicating Hydrocele | Communicating Hydrocele | Hydrocele of the Cord |

When the testicles descend from a baby's abdomen into their scrotum, they are accompanied by a part of the abdominal wall lining. Normally, this abdominal wall lining will break off completely and reconfigure itself to be a sac that surrounds and cushions the testicle. However, In 1–2 percent of males this sac will become filled with fluid, leading to an anatomical condition called a **hydrocele**.

A hydrocele in and of itself is rarely a concern. Most hydroceles will resolve on their own by 1 year of age. However, if a hydrocele is persistent past 1 year of life, it may require surgery to be corrected.

While the hydrocele itself can be mildly discomforting, the main concern with a persistent hydrocele is that it can signal the presence of a persistent pathway between the abdomen and the scrotum. If this pathway does not completely close up and remains intact, it becomes a risk factor for a hernia to occur in the future.

Essentially, a **hernia** is when the intestines escape their normal home—where they should be confined by the abdominal walls. A persistent tunnel from the abdomen to the scrotum provides a perfect setup for the intestines to migrate down into the scrotum. A hernia is a serious concern, and therefore all persistent hydroceles should be evaluated properly by a pediatric surgeon or pediatric urologist.

HYPOSPADIAS

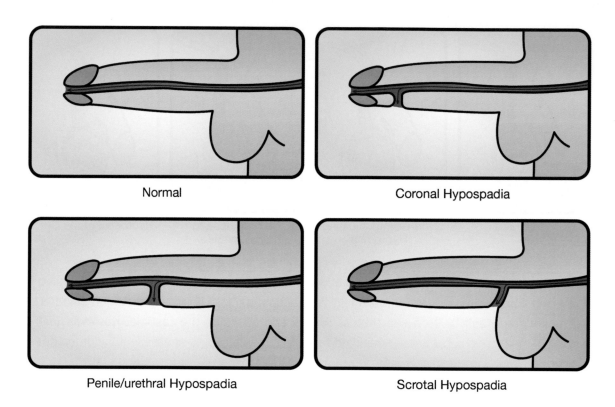

Normal

Coronal Hypospadia

Penile/urethral Hypospadia

Scrotal Hypospadia

About 0.3–0.7 percent of boys will develop a **hypospadias**, which is a condition where the normal opening of the penis (that urine comes out of) is found at an abnormal anatomical location. A hypospadias can be located anywhere along the lower part of the penis. There may be a single hole that is abnormally located, or there may be two openings (with one in the normal position and a second located at an abnormal position).

A hypospadias is often accompanied by other anatomical defects such as a **chordee** (which is where the penis is abnormally curved) and/or an abnormal appearance of the foreskin. A hypospadias should be evaluated by a surgeon (although very mild cases may not require any surgical intervention).

In general, if a hypospadias is found, circumcision should be delayed until a proper evaluation has been completed by a surgeon. Often, the hypospadias correction and circumcision can be done at the same time.

SACRAL DIMPLE

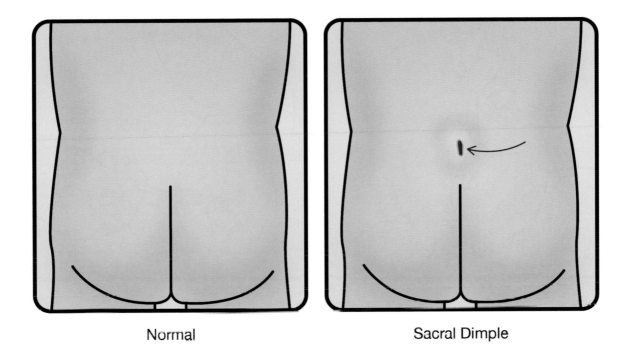

Normal   Sacral Dimple

Sacral dimples are small indentations noted at the upper portion of the buttocks crease. They are quite common and generally benign as long as they are smaller than 0.5 centimeters and the bottom of the dimple is clearly visible.

If the dimple is greater than 0.5 centimeters in size, deep in appearance, has an associated tuft of hair, or shows noticeable skin discoloration, there is a risk that there may be an associated underlying abnormality. Examples include:

- **Spina Bifida**: The mildest version of spina bifida, known as spina bifida occulta, is where the spine does not completely close properly around the spinal cord, but the skin above the spinal cord is intact. In most cases, there are no symptoms.

- **Tethered Cord Syndrome**: The spinal cord is supposed to hang freely in the spinal canal, but at times, the spinal cord can be abnormally tied down, limiting its movement. This can lead to weakness, numbness, muscle issues, and bladder/bowel incontinence.

If a sacral dimple appears unusual, an ultrasound of the spinal cord can help ascertain whether a spinal abnormality is present or not. If any abnormality is seen on ultrasound, a surgical consultation will be necessary.

GAS

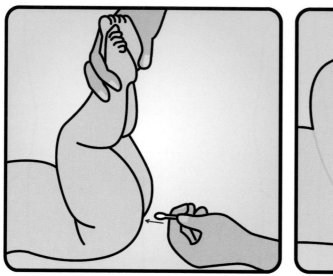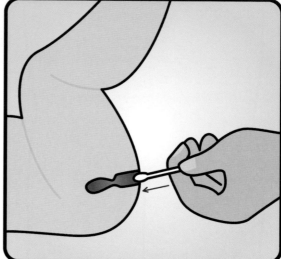

Some of the most common questions that new moms ask are related to gas: how it is made, how to relieve it, why there is so much of it, how can it smell so bad, etc. The good news is that gas is never a danger, but it *is* often a comfort issue.

For the digestive tract to work optimally, there are several components that need to function properly:

- **Peristalsis**: This is the forward-moving, wave-like motion of the intestinal tract that propels food from the mouth to the anus.

- **Enzymes**: The intestines secrete a potpourri of different enzymes to help break down foods.

- **Healthy Gut Bacteria**: When you are first born, your intestines are a blank slate. They are colonized with healthy bacteria over time, which aid in the digestive process.

When babies are first born, the digestive tract needs some time to mature, warm-up, and be colonized with healthy bacteria. This process can take 3–4 months. Until optimal performance is reached there will be quite a lot of gas—up to 20 times a day or more! Even after optimal performance is reached there will still be a lot of gas, but it should not be as painful or quite as plentiful.

Parents will often try different methods to cut down on gaseous emissions: different bottles (to minimize swallowed air), simethicone, homeopathic gas drops, probiotics, formula changes, and different massaging/exercise techniques, to name a few. Unfortunately, there are

What to Know Before Having Your Baby

few studies that show that anything works well. Everything listed is relatively safe—although homeopathic medications are unregulated and probiotics are not fully proven to work for infant gas issues—and thus, while it is reasonable to give them all a try, expectations should be held in check.

The good news is that this, too, shall pass—again, usually around 3–4 months of age. Often, whatever method the parents are employing at 3 months of age is deemed the magic elixir, only to be debunked when the same method fails with the next baby.

One thing that I *am* a personal believer in is a small Swedish tool called a Windi, which can be purchased on the Internet. It is a small, pliable hollow tube that you can insert into the anus to help separate the walls of the anus to allow gas to pass. A poor man's version of this is to massage the anus for 10–15 seconds with a cotton tip applicator coated in petroleum jelly.

Whatever method you choose to use, may the farts be with you.

Sorry. Couldn't resist.

STOOL

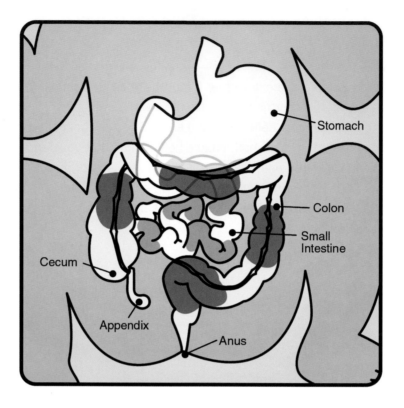

Along with gas issues, the other topic that pediatricians receive a lot of questions about is **poop**. Parents love talking about their baby's poop! A simple guide is this: regardless of the frequency, consistency, color, or smell of your child's stool, if the child is gaining weight and there is no visible blood in the stool, there is little to nothing to be worried about.

Just as we discussed with gas, there will be a change in your child's intestinal tract as they mature. Peristalsis, enzymes, healthy bacteria and what your baby is being fed all contribute to the characteristics of the baby's poop.

Initially, a newborn baby's stool will appear as if you took watery mustard and cottage cheese and mixed the two together. In general, breastfed babies tend to have more watery poops. They also tend to have more frequent poops, with frequency ranging from 10–15 stools a day (one for every feeding) to once every few days. The color of the stool will change regularly to mimic any of the colors of the autumn leaves, while the consistency will range from watery, runny stools to a peanut butter-like texture. And, as the diet changes, so too does the poop.

The bottom line is if your child is gaining weight well, you know they are getting all the nutrition they need. As such, no matter how the stool changes from day to day or week to week, there is little cause for concern.

What to Know Before Having Your Baby

CONSTIPATION

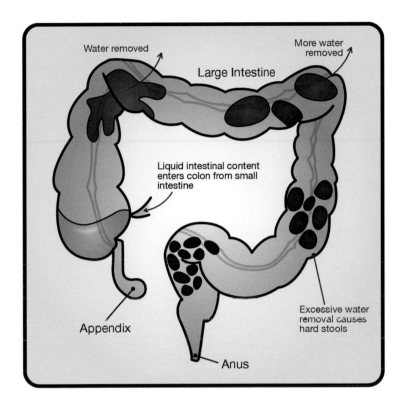

At some point during your baby's first year, they may suffer from **constipation**. Parents often get worried if their child does not produce stool on a daily basis. The truth is, just because your baby does not stool every day does *not* mean they are constipated. After the first few weeks of life, it is perfectly normal for your child to stool once every 2–4 days, or even once a week. It is also perfectly normal for them to strain and grunt (you try pooping laying down!).

Constipation can occur due to three principle reasons:

1. The intestines may be moving too slowly.

2. The intestines may be over-absorbing water from the stool.

3. The stool may not be rich enough in fiber or other water-absorbing food products.

Constipation is better assessed by the thickness of the stool, rather than its frequency. If a child is stooling once a week, but the stool is soft like peanut butter and it comes out easily, there is no need for intervention. No matter the frequency, if the stool is harder than peanut butter and the child is straining, and especially if there is bleeding, intervention may be needed to help soften the stool.

In a normal baby, constipation is for the most part a comfort issue, not a health issue. Rarely does the presence of constipation signal an underlying health issue, but if the child is truly constipated, help is needed to make them more comfortable.

You can start by adding one teaspoon of any type of prune juice to every one ounce of formula or breastmilk, 3–4 times per day. Try this for several days; if this does not work (or your baby is in too much discomfort to wait for this to work), then a visit to the pediatrician is warranted.

DIAPER RASH

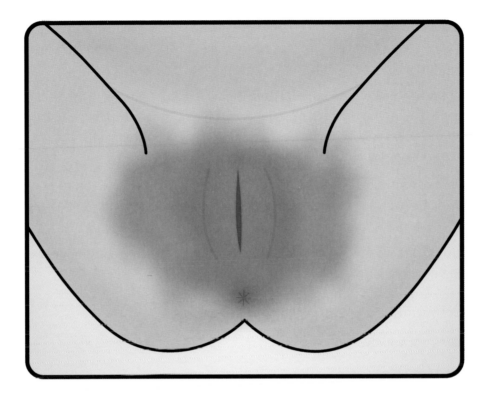

The two most common causes of **diaper rashes** are a chemical irritation rash and a yeast infection.

A **chemical irritation rash** is usually most prominent in the area where the buttocks contact the diaper. The skin can be reddened or severely broken down, and may look like a rug burn or may even be ulcerated.

The other kind of diaper rash is a **yeast infection**, which is caused by a fungus called Candida. Unlike a chemical irritation rash, where the acidity of the stool irritates the skin, a Candida rash is an actual infection that spreads over time until appropriately treated with an anti-fungal cream.

There are two findings that help distinguish a Candida diaper rash from a chemical irritation rash. The first is the presence of the diaper rash in the creases of the skin. Candida will typically affect the creases, whereas a chemical irritation rash will not. The second is the presence of satellite lesions surrounding the diaper rash. The Candida rash will grow in size by shooting out these small satellite lesions from the central base. The satellite lesions will then grow and eventually meld with the central base, expanding the size of the rash over time.

The treatment regimen for all diaper rashes is as follows:

1. **Drying the skin:** Change the diaper as soon as the diaper is soiled or wet. Dry the skin with a blow dryer on a low/cool setting prior to dressing the skin, or alternatively leave the diaper off and allow the skin to "air out" for 5–10 minutes.

2. **Stopping trauma and chemical irritation:** Gently rub stool or urine from the skin with warm water over a sink or tub (instead of using baby wipes). If baby wipes *are* used, rinse out all fragrance and chemicals prior to use by holding them under running warm water for a few seconds, then wringing out the excess water.

3. **Placing a barrier:** Keep a thick barrier in place when the diaper is on to prevent contact with stool and urine while the sensitive skin heals. Any reputable brand of diaper rash cream should work well.

4. **Medications:** If there is a yeast infection, an antifungal cream should be applied underneath the barrier agent with each diaper change.

Please contact your pediatrician if any of the following occur:

- The rash does not improve within a week

- The rash worsens significantly

- Peeling occurs

- Tenderness spreads

- Pus pockets are forming or increasing

- The child develops a fever

PEEING

Feeding & Diaper Goals

Baby's Age	Feeding Frequency	Wet	Stool	Color
Day 1	On-demand (8-12 times / 24 hours)	1	1-2	Greenish-black tarry meconium
Day 2	On-demand (8-12 times / 24 hours)	2	2-3	Greenish-black tarry meconium
Day 3	On-demand (8-12 times / 24 hours)	3	2-3	Brown / green
Day 4	On-demand (8-12 times / 24 hours)	4	2-3	Brown / yellow
Day 5	On-demand (8-12 times / 24 hours)	4+	4+	Yellow
Day 6	On-demand (8-12 times / 24 hours)	4+	4+	Yellow seedy (almost like mustard)
Day 6+	On-demand (8-12 times / 24 hours)	4+	4+	Yellow seedy: some babies switch to less frequent but large bowel movements

Urine output will vary from baby to baby, but some general guidelines can help a family to know what to expect and when to worry.

Day 1: Most likely, your baby will only urinate once during the first 24 hours of life.

Day 2: Your baby will likely urinate twice, and the pee may appear bright yellow as it may be more concentrated.

Day 3: Your baby will likely urinate three times, and the pee will still be bright yellow.

Day 4: Your baby will likely urinate four times, and the pee will begin to lighten a bit in color.

Day 5 and beyond: Expect about 6–8 wet diapers a day.

A good way to remember this pattern is that for the first five days of life, there should be one wet diaper for each day of life. Sometimes it may be hard to count the number of urinations exactly, as the baby may stool and urinate at the same time. As a rule of thumb, if the baby is eating well, is active, and appears well hydrated, then there is little to worry about.

Breastfed babies may have fewer wet diapers in their first few days of life until a mother's milk fully comes in. As long as the baby is active and well hydrated, there is unlikely to be an issue. However, if there is concern for dehydration, a visit to the pediatrician is warranted to discuss feeding options.

URATE CRYSTALS

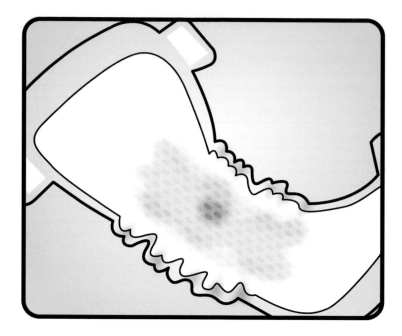

Urate crystals form when calcium and urate combine and crystallize into a reddish-orange byproduct. Both calcium and urate are normal substances in the urine, and the presence of urate crystals is common, especially in newborns.

Although urate crystals are more commonly seen with dehydration, their presence is rarely a cause for concern unless the child is displaying other signs of dehydration, such as diminished activity, poor feeding, or decreased urine output.

Breastfed babies are more likely to display urate crystals in their diaper, especially in the first few days of life when the mother's milk has yet to fully come in. If parents are worried about dehydration, a visit to the pediatrician is warranted; otherwise, the urate crystals should resolve with time.

TAKE-HOME POINTS

★ Hymenal skin tags are small, finger-like protrusions from the vaginal area which are benign and do need to be treated or removed.

★ Labial adhesions appear as a fusion of the skin at the opening of the vagina. Most will resolve on their own with little or no intervention.

★ Many newborn girls will have a whitish or bloody discharge from the vagina caused by hormonal changes. This will resolve on its own within the first few weeks of life.

★ Circumcisions do have multiple health benefits, including significantly lower risk of acquiring sexually transmitted infections and a lower risk of urinary tract infections during the first year of life. Circumcisions heal promptly within a week and can be cared for with regular Vaseline applications with each diaper change until the skin heals.

★ In a small percentage of males, the testicles are undescended at birth, with 70 percent descending on their own by 1 year of age. For those that do not descend on their own, surgical correction is recommended.

★ A hydrocele is a fluid-filled sac next to the testicle that is present in 1–2 percent of newborn males. Most will resolve by 1 year of age, but for those that persist, surgical correction may be recommended.

★ A hypospadias describes a condition in which the normal opening of the penis where urine comes out is found at an abnormal anatomical location. Depending on the severity, surgical correction may be necessary.

★ Sacral dimples are small indentations, noted at the upper portion of the buttocks crease. If the dimple is greater than 0.5 centimeters in size, appears deep, has an associated tuft of hair, or shows noticeable skin discoloration, there is a risk that there may be an associated underlying abnormality.

★ As a newborn's gut matures in the first few months of life, it will produce a lot of gas. Unfortunately, most remedies are not too helpful, but know that this, too, shall pass.

★ A good rule of thumb for newborn stooling patterns is that regardless of the frequency, consistency, color, or smell, if the child is gaining weight and there is no visible blood in the stool, there is little to nothing to be worried about.

★ Constipation is better assessed by the thickness of the stool rather than the frequency of the stool. For the most part, in a normal baby constipation is a comfort issue, not a health issue.

★ Airing out the diaper area with each change will help diaper rashes to heal faster. When a Candida fungal infection is present, an antifungal cream will be necessary.

★ A newborn's urine output for the first five days of life should follow the pattern such that the baby has the same number of wet diapers per day as the number of days they are old. For example, a three-day-old should pee about three times in one day.

★ Urate crystals form when calcium and urate combine and crystallize into a reddish-orange byproduct in the diaper. It is often mistaken as blood, but it is rarely a cause for concern.

What to Know Before Having Your Baby

Chapter 6

ARMS AND LEGS

A S YOUR baby grows, it is fun to see them interact with the world by grabbing their favorite toy, taking their first step, and of course, giving you your first well-deserved hug. As they walk towards you, arms outstretched, you may notice that they start on their tiptoes, or walk bow-legged like a cowboy. This will improve as they develop and their bones straighten out and their gait matures, but it can still be quite concerning for new parents.

Not to worry! Soon they will be running to you for hourly hugs and kisses. All the same, knowing what to expect—and what to watch out for—can go a long way towards putting new parents at ease.

BLUE/COLD HANDS AND FEET

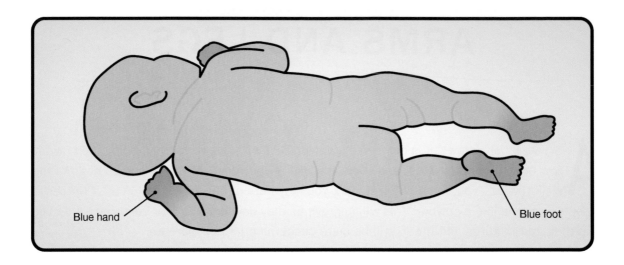

Blue hand

Blue foot

From time to time, you may notice your baby's hands and feet having a **bluish hue** to them. The limbs may also feel cold to the touch compared to the rest of the body. This is quite common in newborns, and their hands and feet should return to a normal pink color as soon as they are warmed up. You may also notice the face, tongue, and lips turning slightly blue when the baby has a good cry, but once they have calmed down, the color will quickly return to normal.

If the blueness is persistently present, however, especially in the facial or torso area, this may be a sign that the heart and lungs are not working properly. Other signs of poor oxygenation include poor feeding, shortness of breath, and the inability to suck for more than a few minutes at a time. If there is concern about oxygenation, an immediate visit to the pediatrician is warranted.

What to Know Before Having Your Baby

DEVELOPMENTAL DYSPLASIA OF THE HIPS

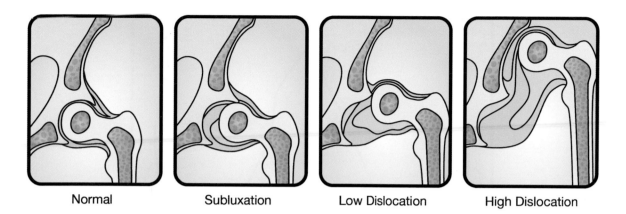

| Normal | Subluxation | Low Dislocation | High Dislocation |

Developmental dysplasia of the hips (DDH) is a dislocation of the hip joint, and when it happens, it will be present at birth. It can affect just one hip or both hips at the same time.

Your normal hip is a ball and socket joint, with the ball portion of the leg bone fitting snugly in the socket portion of the hipbone. If this joint does not form properly, the ball can slip in and out of the socket joint, leading to hip pain and future walking issues.

The reason for DDH is unclear. However, several risk factors make it more likely, including: family history; being a firstborn child; female gender; low amniotic fluid in the uterus; and breech presentation. One theory is that poor positioning of the legs or any stressor giving less room for the hip joint to mature while the infant is in the uterus can lead to a higher risk of the joint not developing properly.

The hips should be examined by the pediatrician at well child checks during the first year of life. If any unusual physical exam findings are noted or if there is a strong history of risk factors, radiological tests or a visit to the pediatric orthopedic doctor is warranted. DDH can be diagnosed with an ultrasound or x-ray depending on the age of the infant.

If caught early, DDH can be treated conservatively with harnesses, which hold the hips in a fixed position, giving the hip joint extra time to fully mature. In more difficult cases, casting or surgery may be necessary. The good news is, if DDH is properly treated, there is an excellent chance of full recovery.

TIBIAL TORSION

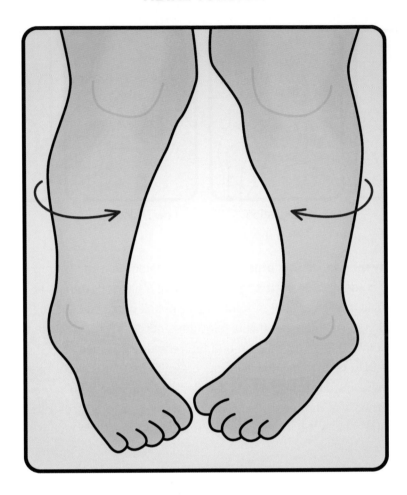

Internal tibial torsion is where the shin bone is abnormally rotated, giving the lower half of the leg a half-moon appearance. It is the most common cause of in-toeing or "pigeon toes" in young children. Parents may notice the condition at birth, but more commonly, they will appreciate it when the child begins walking.

Two-thirds of cases will involve both legs; in the cases where only one leg is affected, the left side is more commonly rotated. It is often associated with and accentuates a bow-legged stance.

The good news is that in most healthy children tibial torsion will naturally improve on its own until 5–8 years of age. If there is still noticeable tibial torsion at 8 years of age, especially if it interferes with walking and running, surgical intervention may be necessary; however, this is rare. Special shoes and braces are not recommended as studies have found them to be ineffective.

What to Know Before Having Your Baby

CLUB FOOT

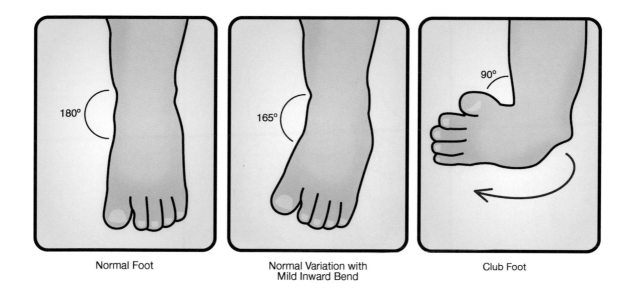

Normal Foot

Normal Variation with Mild Inward Bend

Club Foot

Your body's muscles connect to your bones with connective tissue called **tendons**. If the tendons in the feet are shorter than normal, the foot is placed at an awkward angle. A **club foot** presents as a foot bent inwards, sometimes as severe as 90 degrees or more.

A club foot is more common in males by a two-fold margin. In 30–60 percent of cases both feet are affected. Although genetics and certain conditions in the womb (such as decreased amniotic fluid) can increase the risk of having a club foot, in 80 percent of cases there is no clear cause.

The good news is that a club foot will not cause pain to the baby and there are excellent treatment options. A pediatric orthopedic doctor should be consulted to see which treatment option is the best fit. The typical first line treatment is to cast the affected foot (feet) and gradually move the foot into the correct position. If conservative treatment does not work, surgery may be necessary.

Even with treatment, total correction may not be achievable; however, most children grow up wearing normal shoes and living healthy, active lives.

JOINT CLICKING

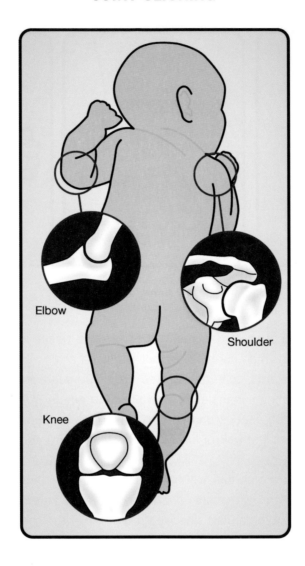

No one knows for sure why joints **click**, but it happens to all of us—babies, children, and adults alike. Theories range from our ligaments stretching and releasing to the compression of gas bubbles in our joint spaces.

Babies will commonly have joint clicking in their knees, shoulders, and elbows. This is all normal and there is no need to worry. However, if the clicking appears to be coming from the infant's hip, it should be evaluated by their pediatrician, as this may be a sign of developmental dysplasia of the hips (see page 85) and may require some radiological tests or a referral to a pediatric orthopedic doctor.

What to Know Before Having Your Baby

TOE WALKING

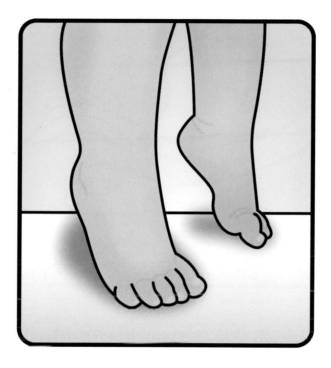

When children begin walking, many will start by walking on their toes or on the balls of their feet. This is known as **toe walking**. This is a common phenomenon and most will outgrow it as they mature. A small percentage of toddlers will continue to walk on their toes out of habit, but even this is rarely a cause for concern. If the child is otherwise developing and growing normally, and especially if you notice that the child walks normally when they are wearing shoes and only toe walks when barefoot, there is little cause for concern.

Most children will outgrow toe walking by 2 years of age. However, toe walking *can* sometimes occur as the result of a nerve or muscle disease such as cerebral palsy or muscular dystrophy. If there are other signs of developmental issues such as unusually tight leg muscles, stiffness in the Achilles tendon, or a general lack of coordination, a visit to the pediatrician is warranted.

NAILS

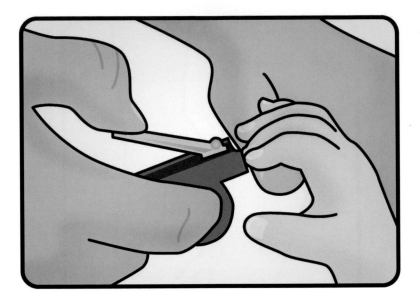

Clipping your baby's **nails** can be a bit unnerving the first time you do it, but you will quickly get the hang of it. A baby's nails grow rapidly and will have to be trimmed at least once a week, if not more frequently. It is important to keep your baby's nails short, as they are prone to scratching themselves and others inadvertently.

You can use a baby nail clipper or baby nail scissors (with rounded tips) to trim the nails. Make sure you have a firm grip of your infant's hands. Sometimes working with a partner can help—one person to hold the baby and the other to focus on trimming the nails. If you are concerned about cutting the baby's skin, you can alternatively use an emery board to file the nails down instead.

Some grandmothers will recommend you initially trim the infant's nails by biting them shorter with your teeth. As your teeth are very sensitive, they can sense just how far to go, and so this method can be safely used. Whichever method you use, the process will get easier as their fingers and toes get bigger!

TAKE-HOME POINTS

★ Blue hands and feet (which may feel cold to the touch) are quite common in newborns and should return to a normal pink color as soon as they are warmed up.

★ Developmental dysplasia of the hips presents when the hip joint does not form properly and can lead to hip pain and future walking issues. If caught early, it can be treated conservatively with harnesses rather than surgery.

★ Internal tibial torsion presents when the shinbone is rotated, giving the lower half of the leg a half moon appearance. In most healthy children, tibial torsion will naturally improve on its own until 5–8 years of age.

★ A club foot is a newborn defect in which the foot appears to be bent inwards, sometimes as severe as 90 degrees or more. All club feet should be evaluated by an orthopedic doctor for treatment.

★ Joint clicking is common, not just in babies, but in all of us. Babies will commonly have joint clicking in their knees, shoulders, and elbows; this is normal and there is no need to worry.

★ A small percentage of children will walk on their toes rather than the balls of their feet. Most children will outgrow toe walking by 2 years of age.

★ Baby's nails grow rapidly and will have to be trimmed at least once a week with a baby nail clipper, baby nail scissors, an emery board, or with the parent's teeth.

Chapter 7

FIRST 2 MONTHS

YOUR FIRST 2 months will be a busy time, with many visitors wanting to meet the baby and the first round of shots being administered. One of the keys to a baby's health will be getting all of their immunizations in a timely manner. Each vaccine has been tested and honed and the schedule that the Center for Disease Control (CDC) recommends is based on decades of data.

Taking a few prudent precautions can help reduce risk and help your baby to avoid unnecessary fever work-ups and minimize exposure to scourges such as whooping cough. By keeping current with their vaccines, and by protecting them with herd immunity, parents can help ensure a healthy beginning and future.

VISITORS IN THE FIRST SIX WEEKS/IMMUNE SYSTEM DEVELOPMENT

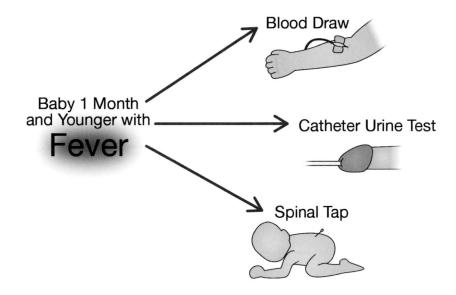

Now that your new baby has come home, it is only natural to want to show them off! However, there are some **precautions** parents should take to avoid the need for further tests and hospitalization. The fact is, new babies show very few signs when they are sick. As such, it is hard to distinguish between a simple viral cold and a dangerous case of bacterial meningitis. Additionally, **when they are first born, babies are more susceptible to serious infections**, owing to the immaturity of their body.

Because of these factors, any new baby (under 4–6 weeks of age) who has a true fever of 100.4°F or higher will require hospitalization and a series of tests, including a blood draw, a catheter urine test, and a spinal tap. Cultures will be sent out to ascertain whether a bacterial infection is present or not in any of the fluids, and will take 48 hours to determine results. Until the cultures are complete, the baby should receive intravenous antibiotics.

This entire process can be harrowing for the parents, but it *is* necessary. Approximately 12 percent of babies with this type of true fever will end up having a serious, possibly life-threatening infection. Granted, this means that 88 percent of babies became febrile from a non-serious illness such as the common cold; nonetheless, it is highly recommended, because of the odds, that all children who present with true fever undergo the full set of tests to check for a serious infection.

To avoid both the threat of a serious infection or the need for a gamut of tests to rule out a serious infection, it is safest to reduce the risk of exposure to germs (by limiting visitors) in the first 4–6 weeks of life. If you want to be extremely conservative, you could extend this out to 12 weeks of life, but this is typically not recommended.

RECTAL TEMPERATURE

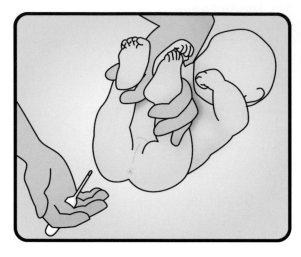 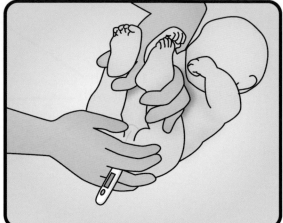

For babies younger than 3 months of age, the best place to check their temperature is in the **rectum** (any thermometer designed for taking rectal temperatures is appropriate). For babies older than 3 months, other methods are reasonable. Often, when parents measure the baby's temperature somewhere other than the rectum, they feel they should add or subtract a degree; however, it is best to report it as shown by the thermometer.

Noting when the temperature was taken, where the temperature was measured, and when the last time a fever-reducing medication was administered can also be useful information. A simple chart documenting these items can also be very helpful.

In children 1 year and older, activity level is a better gauge for how sick a child truly is. For that reason, precise temperature measurements are not as important in older children. Any modality of thermometers is reasonable, and vigilant temperature checking is generally not needed.

How to take a rectal temperature:

1. Lubricate the tip of the thermometer with a lubricating jelly.

2. Lay the baby down (facing up) on a firm flat surface, such as a changing table.

3. Grab the baby's legs securely with one hand.

4. Place the thermometer firmly between the second and third fingers of the free hand.

What to Know Before Having Your Baby

5. Insert the lubricated thermometer through the anal opening, about ½–1 inch (about 1.25–2.5 centimeters) into the rectum. Stop at less than ½ Inch (about 1.25 centimeters) if you feel any resistance.

6. Steady the thermometer between your second and third fingers as you cup your hand against your baby's bottom. Soothe your baby and speak to them quietly as you hold the thermometer in place.

7. Wait until you hear the appropriate number of beeps or any other signal indicating that the temperature is ready to be read. Read and record the number on the screen, noting the time of day that the reading was taken.

HERD IMMUNITY

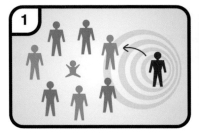
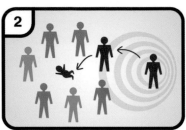
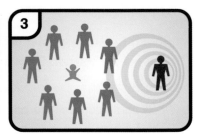

If only SOME get vaccinated, the germ spreads and infects the infant

If ALL get vaccinated, the germ is contained and the infant is safe

Healthy, non-vaccinated   Healthy, vaccinated   Non-vaccinated, sick, contagious

A child's vaccine schedule starts at birth, when they receive the first hepatitis B vaccine. The baby will then receive multiple immunizations at 2, 4, and 6 months. In the first few months of life (until the vaccines produce protective immunity), the infant is vulnerable to many diseases. Furthermore, certain vaccines (particularly the live virus vaccines and the **flu vaccine**) cannot be given until the child is older, which delays protection against these illnesses as well.

Thus, it is important in the first few months of life to promote **herd immunity** until all the important vaccines are given. Herd immunity means that all caretakers who interact with the baby regularly have received vaccines against diseases to which the baby is susceptible, protecting the infant from being exposed to those specific germs.

In the United States, the **DTaP booster** (for whooping cough protection) and the flu vaccine are probably the most important vaccines to receive for the purposes of herd immunization. Other vaccines to consider are hepatitis A, MMR (Measles/Mumps/Rubella), and chicken pox (Varicella). The better immunized a family is, the less risk there is to the infant until they acquire their own protection through the CDC immunization schedule.

Herd immunity is absolutely essential for infants, but it is equally vital for individuals in our society with weakened immune systems, whether it be from cancer treatment, a hereditary condition, or an infection. The ideal way for individuals with weak immune systems to be protected is for those of us with normal immune systems to stay vigilant in receiving vaccines.

PERIODIC BREATHING

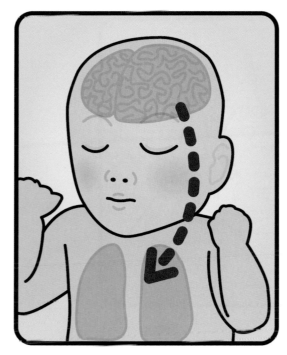

The brain sends signals to the lungs which controls breathing. Periodic breathing happens when the signals are not steady.

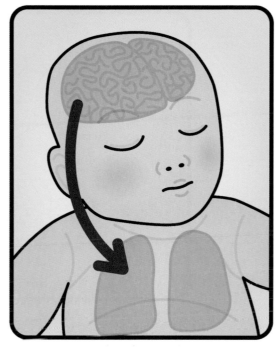

As your baby matures, the signals will become more steady and breathing will be more even and consistent.

Periodic breathing is a normal variation of respiration that can occur in newborns and adults alike. While the baby is breathing normally, the parent may notice a sudden pause in breathing that lasts for no more than 10 seconds, followed by a series of rapid, shallow breaths. Periodic breathing is more prone to happen during deep sleep; however, parents may notice it anytime, even when the baby is fully awake.

Periodic breathing is not a cause for alarm or a sign of a more serious underlying health issue. Up to 80 percent of all infants will display periodic breathing at some time or another. If parents are noticing longer periods of breathing cessation lasting greater than 20 seconds or there are noticeable blue color changes, they should bring it to the attention of their pediatrician as soon as possible.

MORO REFLEX

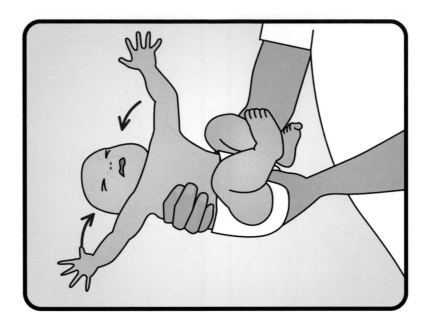

The **Moro reflex**, first described by Austrian pediatrician Ernst Moro, is a sudden outward spreading of the arms, followed by a quick inward embracing motion, usually accompanied by crying. It typically happens in response to a sudden stimulus such as a loud noise, or by dropping the baby 5–10 centimeters through space.

This is a perfectly natural reflex—in fact, it is believed to be one of only a few "unlearned" (or inborn) fears in newborns. You will likely see your infant exhibit this behavior during their first 4–5 months; however, if they continue to demonstrate the Moro reflex much past 6 months of age, you may wish to have them evaluated by their pediatrician.

COLIC

Theories of Colic
Trapped Gas
Gastroesophageal Reflux
Milk Protein Allergy
Lactose Intolerance
Food Allergy
Immature Nervous System
Maternal Anxiety
Bacterial Imbalance

The broad definition of **colic** is 3 hours or more of crying per day, occurring three days a week or more in an otherwise healthy infant who is less than 3 months of age. It is important to note that studies have shown that all babies, whether deemed colicky or not, cry more during the first 3 months of life than at any other time. Approximately 8–40 percent of babies meet the definition of colic. Research has not shown a difference in the incidence of colic between male and female babies, breastfed or formula-fed babies, or between term and preterm infants.

Research has not established the cause of colic. The three main groups of theories are that colic is a manifestation of a gastrointestinal problem, a biological phenomenon, or a psychosocial issue. It may even be some combination of the three categories. Gastrointestinal theories, which are the most popular, include faulty feeding techniques, cow's milk protein intolerance, lactose intolerance, gastrointestinal immaturity, intestinal hypermotility, or alterations in the healthy bacteria of the intestines.

Regardless of the cause of colic, it is clear that colic is not dangerous and will eventually resolve with time. However, excessive crying can be a sign that a more serious issue may be bothering the baby, and as such, an initial evaluation of the infant by your pediatrician can help ascertain whether there are other problems aside from colic.

Once a diagnosis of colic is made, your pediatrician may recommend several interventions to help alleviate crying. Changing feeding techniques or utilizing soothing maneuvers is typically the first line of treatment. Soothing techniques that may help include a pacifier, car rides, rocking, an infant swing, a warm bath, and rubbing the infant's belly. Unfortunately, nothing is a magic quick fix and there is no guarantee that any of the techniques will work.

A slew of other remedies may be recommended by your Aunt Bertha or the Internet at large, such as dietary changes, probiotics, massages, simethicone, herbal remedies, essential oils, and homeopathic remedies. None of these have been proven to work and are not recommended at this time.

The good news is that colic has not been linked to any type of developmental issues and will typically improve by the third month of life. Probably the most important thing is for parents to seek support from friends and family, and when necessary, take a break to refuel. And remember—this, too, shall pass.

What to Know Before Having Your Baby

IMMUNIZATIONS AND ACETAMINOPHEN

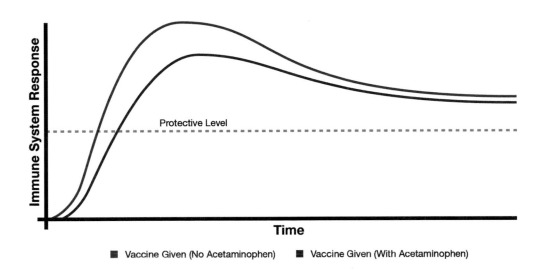

It is common practice to give **acetaminophen** or **fever reducers** to infants when they receive vaccines to reduce the discomfort and pain of receiving immunizations. In 2009, in the Czech Republic, a study was completed looking at the effect acetaminophen has on the body's response to immunizations, both in terms of fever and how the acetaminophen affected the immune system's response to the vaccines.

Not surprisingly, 40–50 percent fewer infants presented with temperatures of 100.4°F or higher in the group who received acetaminophen, as compared to the group who did not receive acetaminophen. Higher temperatures (greater than 103.1°F) were rarely seen in either group and occurred in no more than 1 percent of all children—and to be clear, there was no harm associated with the higher temperatures.

However, although acetaminophen reduced the frequency of fever quite effectively, it also clearly diminished the immune system's response to the vaccines administered. Bear in mind that the purpose of immunizations is to stimulate the immune system to create favorable antibodies to help combat future illnesses. In the group that received acetaminophen, there was a quantifiable decrease in the amount of antibodies produced for several (but not all) of the vaccines given. Ultimately, the vast majority of infants developed protective level of antibodies whether they received acetaminophen or not; however, the group receiving acetaminophen *did* have lower responses.

It is unknown if this decrease in antibody production is clinically significant. It is also unknown whether ibuprofen or other fever reducing agents could produce the same effect—this author's guess is that there is a high probability of this.

Given the Czech Republic study, it is safe to say that it is probably better not to give any acetaminophen when children receive immunizations, if at all possible. Parents may be better off soothing with cold compresses, swaddling, and a pacifier. However, should the child become inconsolable after vaccines it is still reasonable to give them a dose of acetaminophen, as needed, as they should still develop an appropriate level of protection.

IMMUNIZATION SIDE EFFECTS

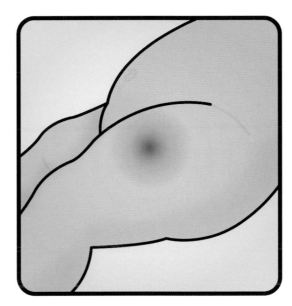

Swelling and Redness

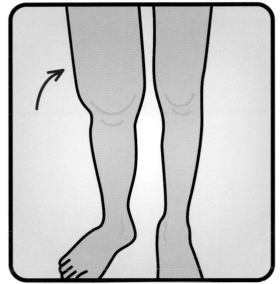

Swollen Leg Syndrome

After your child receives their vaccines. it is quite common for there to be **side effects**. The most common side effects are pain, swelling, and redness at the site of injection. This can be treated with a cold compress applied to the area for 15–20 minutes every hour as needed. Fever is also common and will be seen in 20–33 percent of all children after certain shots. As described previously in this book, it is reasonable to use a fever reducer to help soothe a child, but when possible other measures of comfort should be utilized. At times, you may also notice some localized hives surrounding the area of injection. This can be treated with hydrocortisone 1 percent applied twice a day as needed.

About 1 in a million doses of vaccines could lead to a severe allergic reaction that requires immediate medical attention. If your child breaks out in hives, has swelling of the face and throat, or difficulty breathing, a pediatrician should be contacted right away. Luckily, these types of reactions are few and far between.

Each individual vaccine also has their own potential side effects, none of which are very common. With any vaccine, the benefits of the immunization are always weighed against the potential side effects before they are approved for widespread use.

One common side effect seen with the DTaP (Diphtheria, Tetanus, and acellular Pertussis) vaccine that bears mentioning is swelling of the entire arm or leg for 1–7 days, usually following the fourth or fifth dose of the immunization (typically at 4 years of age). While this can be scary for the family, the side effect is benign and will improve with time without any treatment. Cold compresses can be used for soothing as needed. Most children will be able to move their leg or arm normally, and future DTaP immunizations can still be given, as this is not a true allergic reaction.

What to Know Before Having Your Baby

DEVELOPMENTAL CHARTS

PHYSICAL DEVELOPMENT	Average age skills begin	3 months	6 months	9 months	1 year	2 years	3 years	5 years
Head and trunk control	Lifts head part way up	Holds head up briefly; Holds head up high and well	Holds up head and shoulders; Turns head and shifts weight	Holds head up well when lifted	Moves and holds head easily in all directions			
Rolling		Rolls belly to back	Rolls back to belly	Rolls over and over easily in play				
Sitting		Sits only with full support; Sits with some support	Sits with hand support	Begins to sit without support	Sits well without support	Twists and moves easily while sitting		
Crawling and walking		Begins to creep	Scoots or crawls	Pulls to standing	Takes Steps; Walks	Runs; Can walk on tiptoe and on heels	Walks easily backward	Hops on one foot
Arm and hand control	Grips finger put into hand	Begins to reach towards objects	Reaches and grasps with whole hand	Passes object from one hand to another		Grabs with thumb and forefinger; Easily moves fingers back and forth from nose to moving object		Throws and catches ball
Seeing	Follows close object with eyes	Enjoys bright colors/shapes	Recognizes different faces	Eyes focus on far objects	Looks at small things/pictures		Sees small shapes clearly at 6 meters	
Hearing	Moves or cries at a loud noise	Turns head to sounds; Responds to mother's voice		Enjoys rhythmic music	Understands simple words	Hears clearly and understands most simple language		

Parents like to follow the development of their child by using **charts** that indicate when certain milestones should be met. Often, when certain milestones are not met on time, it produces an anxiety over whether there may be a medical or genetic problem in their child.

The good news is that it is rare for *any* baby to precisely follow the developmental chart in all categories, and most "delays" will correct themselves in due course with watchful waiting. At some point in time, many children will display a temporary delay in their gross motor skills, fine motor skills, speech, or social development. Each child will grow and develop in their unique and individual way, and will often reward a parent's patience just when they think the doctor needs to be seen.

When there is an obvious delay in any category by 2–3 months or more, especially if there is an appreciable delay in multiple developmental categories, it should be brought up to the pediatrician for possible investigation or treatment. Developmental delays should not be ignored, but every parent should be prepared for a few milestones not to be hit by the chart's appointed deadline.

TAKE-HOME POINTS

★ For the first 4–6 weeks of life, it is best to limit the newborn's exposure to germs by avoiding public places where too many people may want to hold the baby, such as church, work, and family gatherings.

★ For babies younger than 3 months of age, the best place to check the temperature is in the rectum.

★ Herd immunity is when all of the caretakers who interact regularly with the baby pro-actively receive vaccines against diseases to which the baby is susceptible, protecting the infant from being exposed to those specific germs.

★ Periodic breathing is a normal variation of respirations where there is a sudden pause in breathing for no more than 10 seconds, followed by a series of rapid, shallow breaths.

★ The Moro reflex is a sudden outward spreading of the arms, followed by a quick inward embracing motion, usually accompanied by crying. It is normal and will be outgrown by 4–5 months of age.

★ The broad definition of colic is 3 hours or more of crying per day, occurring 3 days a week or more in an otherwise healthy infant who is less than 3 months of age. Regard-less of the cause of colic, it is clear that colic is not dangerous and will eventually resolve with time, usually by the third month of life.

★ Giving an infant acetaminophen after immunizations reduces the body's beneficial response to vaccines. As such, it is better not to give acetaminophen after vaccines, instead utilizing other soothing mechanisms, unless the child becomes inconsolable.

★ The most common side effects after immunizations are pain, swelling, and redness at the site of injection. This can be treated with a cold compress applied to the area for 15–20 minutes every hour as needed.

★ Each child will grow and develop in their unique and individual way and will often reward a parent's patience just when they think the pediatrician needs to be seen for a developmental issue.

What to Know Before Having Your Baby

Chapter 8

SLEEPING

NOTHING CAN be more fatiguing for parents than dealing with the sleeping issues of a newborn baby. There are numerous books, methods, and philosophies that parents can read about and implement, but the bottom line is that babies do not have a lot going on, and they will get the sleep they need one way or another.

All the same, moving towards a sleep schedule that works for the family can allow mom and dad to get the rest that they need to take the best care of the newborn. During the process of creating a routine, it is important to follow some guidelines to reduce the risk of Sudden Infant Death Syndrome (SIDS). By following some rules of thumb, parents can work towards a safe and sound sleeping routine that will benefit the baby and the family as a whole.

HOW MUCH SLEEP?

Age	Total Nighttime	Total Naptime	Total Sleep Time
0-2 months	Continuous	Continuous	10-18 hours
2 months	9.5 hours	5 hours	14.5 hours
6 months	11 hours	3.5 hours	14.5 hours
12 months	11.5 hours	2.5 hours	14 hours
3 years	11.5 hours	1.5 hours	13 hours

Newborn babies sleep quite a bit, usually waking up every 2–4 hours for feedings. During the first 1–2 weeks of life, frequent nighttime feedings—every 3 hours or so—can help your newborn return back to their birth weight by 10–14 days of age.

Once a baby is back to their birth weight, there is no need to wake a sleeping baby at night to feed them. Breast milk and formula should only be offered when they awaken; a minimum of 3 hours should pass between each feeding and it is best to allow your baby to go as long as they will tolerate between nighttime feeds. Know that awakening your baby to feed them or offering food every time they stir during the night will either start or propagate a habit of waking up to feed.

You may have heard that starting solid foods or adding cereal to their bottle will help a baby sleep through the night. However, there is no evidence this is true. At about 2 months of age, most babies have the ability to start sleeping through the night, although a few cooperative babies may start sooner.

The above table is a guideline as to how much babies sleep. However, each baby is unique and may not follow the table exactly.

CREATING A BEDTIME AND SLEEP ROUTINE

Time	Action
7:15	Taking a bath
7:30	Changing the diaper and changing into pajamas
7:45	Hearing a story or singing a song
8:00	Place in crib

Starting from 4 weeks to 3 months of age (or sooner), you should begin to create a bedtime routine which will signal to your baby that it is time to go to sleep. A routine can include any and all of the following:

• Taking a bath

• Changing the diaper and changing into pajamas

• Hearing a story or singing a song

The baby's own crib away from the parents (if possible). Put your infant to sleep while they are drowsy, but *awake*. Establishing this habit early will teach your child to go back to sleep on their own when they awaken in the middle of the night.

Once you put your baby down in the crib, leave the area as soon as possible. If the baby begins to cry, resist the urge to intervene and allow them to learn to comfort themselves. Even if the crying lasts for several hours it is safe; rest assured, however, that they will likely fall asleep in less than an hour.

Some babies will sleep through the night (10–11 hours continuously) starting as early as 1 month of age, but all babies should be able to do this by 3 months of age. It is okay to feed the baby at night, however try to limit this as much as possible. A 1-month-old should eat no more than twice a night, a 2-month-old should eat no more than once a night, and a 3-month-old should be sleeping 10–11 hours continuously at night. Night is defined as a 10–11 hour period from 8 pm to 6–7 am. Whatever your baby does not eat at night, they will make it up during the day!

For various reasons, throughout the first two years your baby may start to wake up again during the night. Let them stay in their bed, change their diaper if it is dirty or wet (but keep the lights down), and remember that it is okay to let them cry and soothe themselves back to sleep.

Generally, the less intervention the better, and the sooner the waking episodes will be extinguished. Try not to pick your baby up or reintroduce feeding during the night as it may start a habit that will be difficult to break. The pattern of uninterrupted nighttime sleep and peaceful bliss will soon return.

SWADDLING

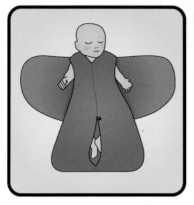

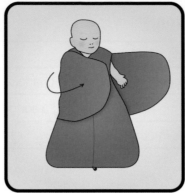

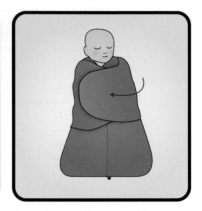

Dress your baby in pajamas. Put your baby's arms through the upper holes. Tuck their feet in and zip up the wearable blanket.

Tuck in each arm and fold the swaddle over the respective arm.

Swaddle should be snug, safely below the chin, and aligned appropriately with the baby's shoulders.

Most parents like to **swaddle** their newborn (wrap them up in some kind of blanket or covering) and when done effectively it can calm infants and help them to sleep. Swaddling carries some risks however—namely **Sudden Infant Death Syndrome (SIDS)** and **developmental dysplasia of the hips (DDH)**.

To reduce the risk of SIDS, once babies are rolling over on their own, swaddling should be discontinued.

To reduce the risk of DDH, parents should watch a video on how to appropriately swaddle a child while keeping the hips loose. If babies are swaddled too tightly, it may increase the risk of DDH, which is previously described in this book. An excellent video on proper swaddling techniques can be found at the website of the International Hip Dysplasia Institute.

What to Know Before Having Your Baby

SUDDEN INFANT DEATH SYNDROME (SIDS)

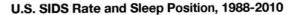

U.S. SIDS Rate and Sleep Position, 1988-2010

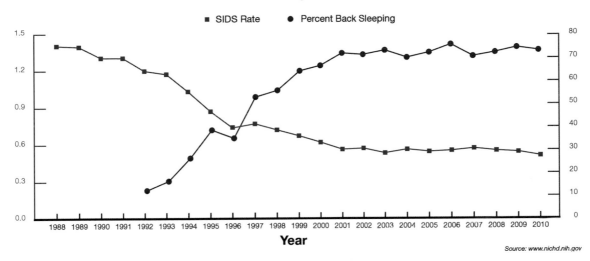

■ SIDS Rate   ● Percent Back Sleeping

Source: www.nichd.nih.gov

Sudden Infant Death Syndrome (**SIDS**) is the leading cause of **infant death** beyond the neonatal period. However, since 1992 when the American Academy of Pediatrics recommended that babies be positioned on their backs while sleeping, the SIDS rate in the United States has decreased by more than 40 percent.

The AAP has made the following recommendations concerning infant sleep:

- Infants should be placed for sleep on their back. Supine (wholly on their back) confers the lowest risk and is preferred.

- Only allow your baby to sleep in a crib that conforms to the safety standards of the Consumer Product Safety Commission and the American Society for Testing and Materials.

- Infants should not be put to sleep on waterbeds, sofas, soft mattresses, or other soft surfaces.

- Avoid soft materials in the infant's sleeping environment (plush blankets, stuffed animals, pillows, or soft bumpers for the crib/bassinet).

- Bed sharing or co-sleeping may be hazardous, especially during the first 4 months of life.

- Overheating should be avoided. The infant should be lightly clothed for sleep, and the bedroom temperature should be kept comfortable for a lightly clothed adult. Over-bundling should be avoided, and the infant should not feel hot to the touch.

- A certain amount of tummy time while the infant is awake and observed is recommended for developmental reasons and to help prevent flat spots on the head. Consider alternating the side of the head the infant sleeps on weekly or daily.

- Sleep positioning devices are not recommended.

- There is no evidence that home apnea monitors decrease the incidence of SIDS.

- A pacifier used during sleep time can decrease the risk of SIDS.

- Once babies are rolling over on their own, swaddling should be discontinued.

- There is some evidence that room-sharing with the infant up to 6–12 months of life (on a separate sleep surface) may reduce the risk of SIDS.

TAKE-HOME POINTS

★ Once a baby is back to their birth weight, there is no need to wake a sleeping baby at night to feed. Feed them only when they awaken; a minimum of 3 hours should pass between each feeding.

★ Ideally, a newborn should be feeding no more than two times a night by 1 month of age; once a night by 2 months of age; and zero times a night by 3 months of age. Night is defined as a 10–11 hour period from 8 pm to 6–7 am.

★ Swaddling should be done properly to give the hips room to move to reduce the risk of developmental dysplasia of the hips (DDH).

★ Swaddling should stop once the baby begins to roll over on their own to reduce the risk of Sudden Infant Death Syndrome (SIDS).

★ Always lay your baby on their back at night and review all of the ways to reduce the risk of Sudden Infant Death Syndrome (SIDS).

Chapter 9

FEEDING

ATING SHOULD be fun! At a scientific level, eating is about getting the right nutrition and keeping the body healthy. But, more broadly speaking, mealtime is an important time of the day for every family to socialize, catch-up, and enjoy good food together. The eventual goal of feeding time is to move the infant towards solid foods, so that by 1 year of age they can eat what the rest of the family is eating and experience healthy eating together!

Bear in mind, feeding children is as much an art as it is a science. There may be many different methods, books, or suggestions that you will encounter, but similar to establishing a sleeping routine, the vast majority of babies will make sure they get what they need one way or another.

As a rule of thumb, the parent is in charge of the **quality** of the food, and the child is in charge of the **quantity** of the food. As long as a well-balanced diet is followed, children will gain the weight they need and optimize their health. By keeping a few tips and concepts in mind, parents and infants can enjoy mealtime even from an early age and make it a highlight of the day.

WHAT TO FEED

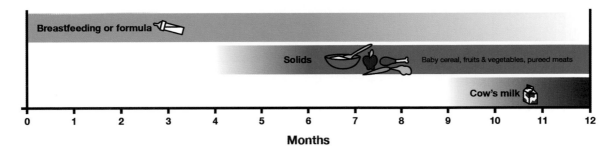

Without exception, **breast milk** is the best food for babies during the first year of life. The American Academy of Pediatrics encourages breastfeeding until 1 year of age. If 1 year seems excessive, pick an alternative goal that is more realistic for you (such as 6 months).

Breast milk provides just the right balance and amount of nutrients that babies need for good growth and development. It also contains substances that help protect babies from certain illnesses, and even reduces the risk of developing allergies and asthma.

If you choose not to breastfeed, you cannot breastfeed, or if you stop nursing before your baby's first birthday, **infant formula** provides an excellent alternative to breast milk. Do not worry or feel guilty if you need to use formula; this author was an exclusively formula-fed infant, as was my younger brother—and we did not turn out too weird!

United States guidelines state that whole milk should not be given until 1 year of age (although some countries recommend starting at 9 months of age, which is reasonable and cheaper!) and reduced fat cow's milk is not recommended until after the second birthday. Compared to breast milk or formula, cow's milk does not supply the balanced nutrition your baby needs and it can be hard on your baby's sensitive digestive system if given too early.

Breast milk and formula normally provide all the water your baby needs. Additional water or juice is not necessary, and could prove harmful due to the immaturity of your newborn baby's kidneys. A baby who is urinating at least six times per 24 hours is not in need of additional fluids. A safe time to start giving plain water is after 4 months of age.

The American Academy of Pediatrics recommends that no solid foods (e.g. rice cereal) be given before 4 months of age. Many parents are eager for the day their baby begins to take solid foods. However, there are several reasons to wait until at least 4 months. If solids are introduced too early, the risk of food allergies and even type-2 diabetes could be increased (however, studies are limited regarding this fact). The extra calories may also make your baby overweight. Additionally, most babies are not able to swallow foods well during the first few months of life, creating a choking hazard. Strictly from a nutritional standpoint, solid foods are not necessary during the first 4–6 months of life. Breast milk and formula provide all the nutrients a baby needs.

WHEN TO FEED

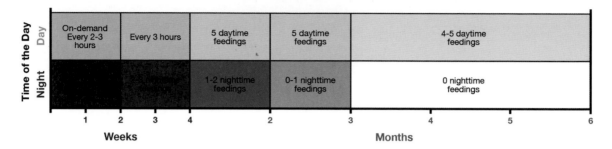

There is a controversy in our culture concerning feeding on-demand versus feeding on a schedule. It is generally more practical to feed on a schedule; filling your baby with each feeding allows for time to play and sleep in between feeds. On the other hand, almost all babies respond well to feeding on-demand, particularly in the first few weeks of life. However, this approach can become quite a drain on mom and quite a strain on her nipples, as babies tend to "demand" feedings quite often. Some moms cannot tolerate feeding on-demand.

Both methods have their advantages and disadvantages, so explore each option to determine which is best for you and your baby. Admittedly, it is this author's bias that a schedule works better for most families in the long run. However, it must be emphasized that some babies cannot easily be put on a schedule in the first few weeks of life. Milk supply constraints and baby feeding abilities sometime require a feed on-demand style; however, with maturity all babies can adopt a schedule eventually.

During the day, you should aim to have your baby eat every three hours, even if this means waking your baby up to feed (although for the first 1–2 weeks, they may require more frequent feeds). During the night, do not wake a sleeping baby to feed (this is safe to do once the baby has regained their weight back to their original birth weight which is usually by 10–14 days of life). They will awaken on their own when they are hungry and whatever they do not get at night they will make up during the day.

Babies should be trained to sleep at night and to feed during the day—despite their tendency to do just the opposite. In general, babies are very reliable at asking for as many calories as they need to grow. Do not worry that you are not giving them enough food; as long as your baby is awakening to feed, has good wet diapers, and is satisfied for 2–3 hours after each feeding, then they are getting enough to eat.

Your new baby may cry as often as every hour. However, keep in mind that babies don't need to be fed every time they cry. They may just feel the need to soothe themselves—so offer a pacifier at that time. Your baby may be protesting that their diaper is wet or that they need a nap. Before you offer the breast or bottle, be sure your baby is not crying for some reason other than hunger.

What to Know Before Having Your Baby

If you see a pattern of hunger soon after feeds, encourage your baby to eat more at each feeding. In addition, you might try to buy a little more time between feeds by using a pacifier as a distraction. Babies have a "non-nutritive" sucking need that is very soothing for them. If breastfeeding has been well established for 2 weeks or longer, you do not have to worry about nipple confusion. When your child cannot be distracted anymore, they will be hungry enough to eat more than before. Usually, the more a baby takes during a feed, the longer they will be content between feeds. Using this method, feeds can be spaced out and a schedule can be created.

It is best not to get into the habit of offering frequent small feedings to please a fussy baby. The offerings might encourage a pattern of frequent, unpredictable snacking instead of more filling feeds that fully satisfy your baby, which can move them closer to a more practical schedule.

Babies differ in their feeding needs and preferences, but by 1 month most breast-fed babies will feed approximately every 3 hours, nursing 10–20 minutes on each breast. Formula-fed babies will usually feed every 3–4 hours and finish a bottle in 30 minutes or less.

Between birth and 1 month of age, gradually move towards a schedule. Some babies will come home and fall into an every 3 hour schedule almost right away. However, most babies will need a good bit of parenting when it comes to simplifying the feeding process. As important as it is to feed your baby, do not forget that you are part of the equation; schedules are important to help keep moms sane and well rested!

HOW MUCH TO FEED

Baby's Age	Formula
First week	1½-3 oz
Month 1	2-3 oz
Month 2	3-4 oz
Month 3	4-6 oz
Month 4	5-7 oz

How can you tell whether your baby is getting enough breast milk or formula? The best confirmation of good nourishment is good weight gain. With each doctor's visit, a weight check will be done and in general babies should gain about ½–1 ounce of weight per day or approximately two pounds per month over the first 4 months of life. Bear in mind that most babies will lose weight the first five days of life before weight gain begins.

That said, your baby may be eating too much if you notice large amounts of spitting-up after feeds. Usually, a baby will stop eating when they are full, but sometimes they will eat a little more than they should. Try smaller volumes more frequently if you suspect overfeeding. Bear in mind that spitting-up is quite normal for most babies and is not always a sign of overfeeding—use your parental judgment on this!

The above table is a guideline as to how much babies eat. However, each baby is unique and may not follow the table exactly.

Signs of a well-fed baby include:

• Happy and satisfied after feedings

• Wets six or more diapers daily (after five days of age)

• Sleeps well between feedings

• Gains weight of ½–1 ounce per day

Most newborns weigh between 5–10 pounds, with the average being about seven and a half pounds. During the first five days of life, infants generally lose 4–10 ounces of weight, with breastfed babies possibly losing a little more. This weight loss is no cause for concern, as it is all part of the baby's adjustment to the outside world. Most of the weight loss is water, and by 14 days of age most babies will gain back what they have lost. Healthy, well-fed babies generally double their weight by 4–5 months and triple their weight by 1 year of age.

SPITTING-UP/REFLUX

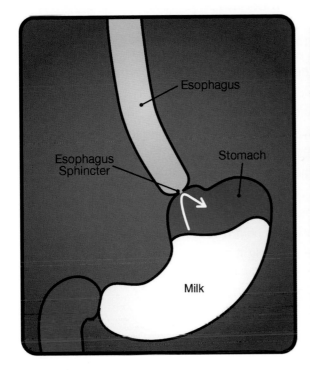
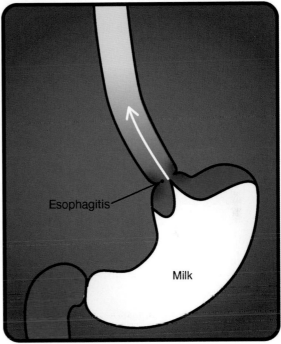

In most babies, **spitting-up** (or **reflux**) is a laundry issue, not a medical issue. We generally refer to frequent mess-makers as "happy spitters". More than 60 percent of all healthy infants will spit-up on a regular basis and the vast majority will not require any medications or serious intervention.

Spitting-up in healthy babies occurs because of the immaturity of their digestive tract. When a baby is first born, their stomach is tiny and not very distensible. Thus, when the infant eats beyond the holding capacity of the stomach, it contracts, forcing food upward and causing the baby to spit-up. However, as kids mature the stomach will grow in size, become more distensible and be able to hold larger amounts of food without spitting-up.

Spitting-up will typically resolve by about 8–12 months of age, but in some children the problem will persist until 18 months or later.

Spitting-up can be concerning if any of the following issues are noted:

- Poor weight gain, especially when the growth curve is not being followed

- Persistent fussiness occurring when the baby is spitting-up, particularly if there is arching of the back

- Bright fluorescent yellow or fluorescent green vomit

- Vomiting blood or stooling blood

- Consistent forceful vomit that shoots out of the mouth like a projectile

If none of the above issues are present, then there is little cause for concern and medications are not needed.

Lifestyle changes that may help include holding the baby upright for 20–30 minutes after feedings, giving smaller feedings more frequently, thickening feeds, and burping halfway between the meal (in addition to at the end of the meal). Formula changes are only helpful if there is a true milk protein allergy (which is not too common); in most happy spitters this is unnecessary and will not make much of a difference.

If a baby displays poor weight gain or is persistently fussy as they spit-up, there may be a benefit to using an acid suppression medication to help treat reflux. For any parent who is worried, a thorough exam by their pediatrician and a weight check can help rule out any serious issues. But in most cases, the only intervention needed is a few extra loads of laundry.

What to Know Before Having Your Baby

BREASTFEEDING

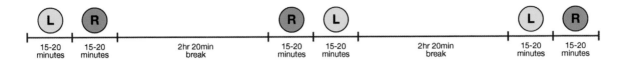

Usually, breast milk does not come in until the fourth day of life. Until then, a clear or yellowish fluid called **colostrum**, which is extra-rich in nutrients and immunity enhancers, will come from your breasts.

At first, your new baby will nurse often (eight or more times in a 24 hour period). But as the breast milk comes in, your baby will get more and more with each feeding and will gradually space out their feeds. You know your baby is getting milk if you can see it in their mouth during the feed and if you can hear them swallowing after every few sucks. Most newborn babies will automatically consume what their body needs within a 24 hour period—they are born with a survival instinct, after all!

During the first couple of weeks, one of the most common issues with breastfeeding is keeping your baby awake during feeds. Gently arousing your baby by moving, burping, and tickling them can help stimulate your baby to feed while on the breast. Some babies feed better if they are naked (except for their diaper).

However, even with the best efforts, some children will choose to sleep rather than feed. Some babies would just sleep and snack all day if we let them, using mom as a human pacifier. In general, keep feeds to less than 45 minutes to prevent maternal exhaustion. Most babies get the largest amount of milk per feed during the first ten minutes on each breast.

With time, the baby and the mom will become more efficient at breastfeeding. The first few weeks of nursing will be a learning period for you and your baby. Neither of you may accomplish a lot on your first few tries, but that's all right. It might be tough, but if you make it through the first few weeks, it *will* get easier!

TENDER NIPPLES

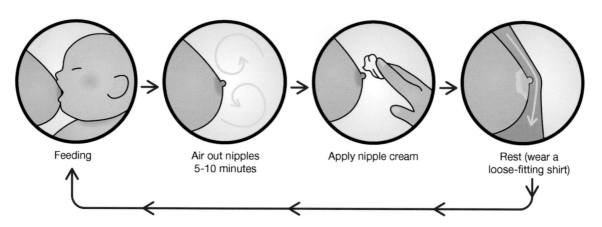

Feeding

Air out nipples
5-10 minutes

Apply nipple cream

Rest (wear a
loose-fitting shirt)

Tender nipples is a common problem when breastfeeding. You can use nipple creams (such as Lanolin) and salt water soaks as needed. More importantly, try to keep the nipples as dry as possible between feeds. They need to be aired out regularly in order to heal. Do not sleep with bras or tight clothing. Try to wear a loose fitting t-shirt during the day, and avoid wearing a bra if possible.

Try not to use breast pads when you have dry, cracked, or sore nipples. In addition, be certain that the pain is not being caused by your baby "latching on" incorrectly (a lactation consultant can help to determine this).

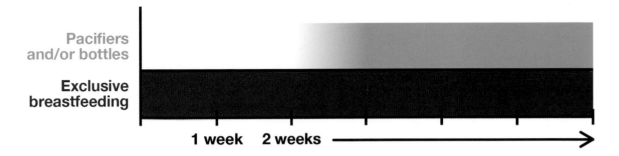

NIPPLE CONFUSION

If you are choosing to breastfeed, you have probably been warned at some point to be wary of using a pacifier or bottle as infants may become "**nipple confused**," which essentially means they begin to prefer the bottle or pacifier over the breast. While there are certainly many anecdotes that back up this phenomenon, the most recent studies indicate that there is probably little to worry about.

If you are choosing to breastfeed, your chances of success are probably the same whether you use supplemental bottles/pacifiers or not. Some studies even show that there is a higher rate of breastfeeding success when supplementing with bottle-feeding. Regardless, it is safe to say that the most likely indicator of success is the mom's determination to breastfeed. Unfortunately, not everyone that *wants* to breastfeed will succeed. However, when problems arise it is usually a supply issue and *not* nipple confusion.

Pacifiers can be a great way to soothe babies and have been shown to decrease the risk of SIDS (Sudden Infant Death Syndrome). Bottle-feeding (either with formula or pumped breastmilk) can help others to get involved with feeding, reducing the burden on mom and providing extra calories when needed, not to mention being more convenient in certain situations.

If there is a high level of concern about nipple confusion, parents can hedge their bets by waiting two weeks until breastfeeding is well established before introducing pacifiers and bottles. Most babies however will be able to handle artificial nipples and breastfeeding harmoniously without too much fuss and trouble.

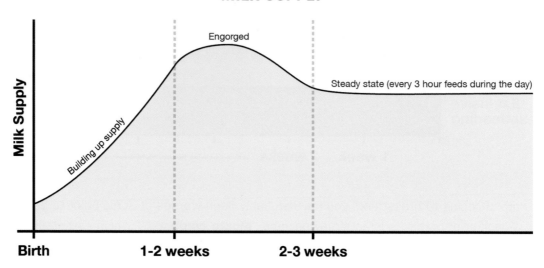

MILK SUPPLY

Engorged

Steady state (every 3 hour feeds during the day)

Building up supply

Milk Supply

Birth   **1-2 weeks**   **2-3 weeks**

Low **milk supply** is a common cause of breastfeeding frustration. Breastfeeding is a "use it or lose it" endeavor; in other words, the breasts must be emptied thoroughly and often enough to build and sustain milk supply (at least every 3–4 hours).

Try to alternate which breast you offer first at each feed. (Some breastfeeding mothers put a safety pin on their bra to remind themselves where to start the next time.) In this way, the breasts will be emptied more evenly and completely.

If your baby cannot effectively empty both breasts, then consider using a pump. Some moms will need to use the pump until their baby is old enough to take large, efficient feeds. Some babies may need supplementation with pumped breast milk or formula given in a bottle.

Pumping not only stimulates milk production, it also enables someone other than mom to feed your baby if necessary. It may be best to hold off on the bottle until breastfeeding is well established (usually after 2 weeks of life). At 2 weeks of age, most babies can take a couple of bottles a day and still continue to breastfeed well. Whether you are breastfeeding directly or pumping, remember that if the breasts are not stimulated and emptied enough, milk supply will decrease.

If it becomes necessary to supplement your breastfeeding to maintain growth, boost urine output, or to completely satisfy your baby, always breastfeed first, then offer the bottle.

As your milk supply increases, your baby should take less and less of the bottle, and eventually you can drop the bottle feedings altogether. However, after breastfeeding is well established, mothers may want to purposefully give a bottle occasionally so that their baby will not refuse a bottle in the future. If a bottle is never introduced, things may become difficult when mom needs to go back to work, go out with dad, or go out of town unexpectedly. An every-other-day bottle should be sufficient enough to maintain bottle feeding proficiency.

WHAT TO EAT WHEN BREASTFEEDING

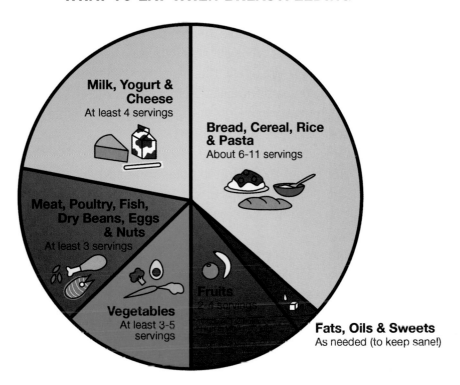

DAILY FOOD GUIDE FOR BREASTFEEDING MOTHERS

Milk, Yogurt and Cheese	At least 4 servings
Meat, Poultry, Fish, Dry Beans, Eggs and Nuts	At least 3 servings
Vegetables	At least 3–5 servings
Fruits	2–4 servings (choose two foods high in vitamin C and folic acid, and one food high in vitamin A)
Bread, Cereal, Rice and Pasta	About 6–11 servings
Fats, Oils and Sweets	As needed (to keep mom sane!)

This is just a guide, and you may need to eat more than this based on your size and activity level.

Most moms will do just fine for breastfeeding following the same diet as their pregnancy. As a nursing mother, you'll need to eat a balanced diet that contains **about 500 calories more per day** than the diet you needed pre-pregnancy.

In general, lactating women should get nutrients from a well-balanced, varied diet, rather than from vitamin and mineral supplements. Eat generous amounts of fruits and vegetables, whole grains and cereals, calcium-rich dairy products, and protein-rich foods (meats, fish, and legumes). For the most part, foods in the mother's diet very rarely have a disturbing effect on their babies. Foods such as tomatoes, onions, cabbage, chocolate, and spicy foods have a reputation for causing gas, and other foods such as milk, soy, eggs, nuts, wheat, and fish have a reputation for causing allergies—but again, this is not too common.

Continue taking your daily prenatal vitamins. Remember, however, that vitamin and mineral supplements do not take the place of food. It is better to get your nutrients from a well-balanced diet than to rely on a vitamin and mineral supplement.

Be sure to drink lots of fluids—at least 6–8 glasses of water a day, approximately one glass for every time you nurse or pump. You need the fluids to replace what you lose through your breast milk. Don't drink more than two cups of coffee, tea, cola, or other caffeine-containing beverages a day; caffeine passes into your breast milk and can make your baby irritable or cause difficulty sleeping.

If your baby has loose stools, blood in their stools, colic, or excess gas for no reason that you can think of, you may review your diet from the previous 24 hours and even consider eliminating some of the foods listed above (milk and soy first) to see if it helps. If you think your baby is reacting negatively to foods that you are eating, especially if there is repeated blood in the stool, discuss this with your pediatrician as soon as possible.

HEALTH RECOMMENDATIONS FOR THE BREASTFEEDING MOTHER

Alcohol	Amount	Clearance Time from Breast Milk
Beer	12 oz	3 hours
Wine	5 oz	3 hours
Liquor (40%)	1.5 oz	3 hours

It is best to **abstain from alcohol** while you are breast-feeding, just as you did during your pregnancy. Alcohol is readily passed into human milk. Any heavy drinking or daily drinking of even small quantities of alcoholic beverages could hurt your baby. If you have a hospitalized, premature or ill newborn and you are breastfeeding, do not drink *any* alcohol. Having said that, an occasional beer or glass of wine is probably safe as long as you wait for the alcohol to completely clear before breastfeeding again (see the above chart).

Do not smoke, as smoking can decrease your milk supply. Also, the breakdown products from nicotine can pass to your baby through your milk. If you cannot stop smoking altogether, try to cut down as much as possible. If you must smoke, do it shortly *after* nursing your baby. Above all, do not smoke in the same room as your baby or even in the house, if possible. Change your shirt before holding them; breathing your exhaled smoke, even the particles on your clothes, can hurt your baby. It can possibly contribute to cancer later in life and can make your baby more at risk for asthma, allergies, and even ear infections.

STORAGE OF BREAST MILK

Location	How Long Breast Milk Can Safely Be Stored For	
	Freshly Expressed Milk	**Thawed Milk**
Room Temperature	4 hours	3 hours
Refrigerator	4-7 days	3 hours
Freezer (compartment inside a refrigerator)	2 weeks	3 hours
Freezer (compartment with a separate door)	3-4 months	3 hours
Separate Deep Freeze	6 months or longer	3 hours

Storing milk in 2–4 ounce amounts (or approximately what is needed for 1–2 feeds) can help with efficiency and reduction of waste. Refrigerated milk has more anti-infective properties than frozen milk, but do not be afraid to freeze when needed. It is best to cool milk in the refrigerator before adding it to already frozen milk if you are combining them into one container. Breast milk, depending on whether it is freshly expressed or thawed, can be stored and used per the above chart.

When you are thawing or heating milk it is not a good idea to use the microwave, as the microwave can denature proteins (meaning it destroys the good stuff in the milk). Also, the microwave can superheat random pockets of milk that can burn your baby's mouth. Instead, warm frozen or refrigerated milk by submersing or running under hot water until it hits the appropriate temperature.

MEDICATIONS WHEN BREASTFEEDING

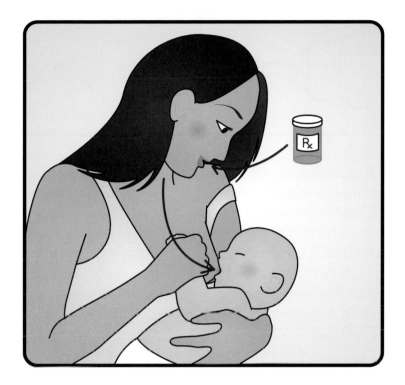

Medications taken by a mother can pass into her breast milk. This applies to both prescription and over-the-counter drugs. The most common medications that can cause problems with breast-feeding babies are sedatives taken for sleep, tranquilizing agents, mood-altering drugs, a few antibiotics, anti tuberculosis medications, chemotherapeutic agents and seizure medications.

Almost all over-the-counter medications are safe in their recommended doses. If you need to take a medication that is compatible with breastfeeding, always take the medication immediately after you complete a feeding. This gives your body several hours to metabolize the medication before the next feeding time and minimizes the amount passed to your baby.

If you ever have questions about the safety of breastfeeding while you are on a certain medication, contact your pediatrician. Medications and a Mother's Milk by Thomas W. Hale is also an excellent resource on the effects of maternal medication on the breastfeeding infant.

BOTTLE FEEDING

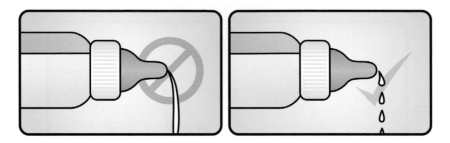

Infant formula or expressed/stored breast milk should be the **only form of milk** your baby gets during the first 9–12 months of life. When your baby comes home from the hospital, they will probably take 1.5–3 ounces of breastmilk or formula at each feeding. When they are able to empty the bottle, you may begin offering more at each feed in order to satisfy them.

Cleanliness is important for small babies, especially when it comes to things that go in their mouths. You'll need to be careful about keeping containers, bottles, nipples, and utensils free of germs. Everything should be washed thoroughly in hot, soapy water and rinsed with plain, hot water similar to washing the dishes. As a rule of thumb, if the cleaning routine is safe for the parent, it is safe for the baby.

You should wash your hands well with soap and water before beginning formula preparation. After each feeding, rinse the bottle and nipple with cool water. If you rinse the milk away before it can form a film, washing will be easier later. There is no reason to sterilize water that is used to prepare the baby's formula. As a rule of thumb, if the water is safe for the parent, it is safe for the baby.

The size of the nipple hole should be large enough to let milk flow freely, one drop at a time. If the milk doesn't form separate drops or flows too fast, throw the nipple away. If the formula flows too slowly, carefully enlarge the nipple hole with a needle or toothpick.

As you feed your baby, keep the bottle tilted so formula fills the nipple and the baby can't suck any air through. Too much swallowed air will give them a false sense of fullness and may lead to discomfort from gas later.

It is perfectly fine to give formula that is room temperature or even cold—warming the formula is based on preference (and similarity to body-temperature breastmilk), and not because of health reasons. Never heat formula in the microwave as it can create pockets of hot formula that can burn the baby's mouth. It is best to warm formula by running the bottle under warm water or placing it in a container with warm water.

While it is important to be clean and follow good habits, there is no need to buy bottle warming machines, special baby water, or top-of-the-line bottles. Babies will be healthy and do just fine by following some sensible routines.

What to Know Before Having Your Baby

FORMULA SELECTION

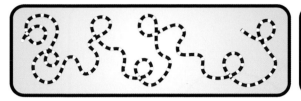

Whole proteins in cow's milk or routine formula.

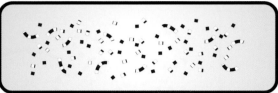

Small protein fragments in an extensively hydrolyzed formula.

Breastfeeding may not make sense for every family, whereas formula provides a convenient, effective alternative. But which formula to purchase?

In some ways, it's hard to go wrong with **formula selection**. All formulas sold in the United States must meet the nutrient standard set by the Food and Drug Administration (FDA). For the most part, the dizzying selection of formulas is a result of marketing, and most babies will do fine in the long run with any formula the parents settle upon.

There are three major groups of formulas available for parents to choose from: **cow milk-based formulas**, **soy-based formulas**, **and protein hydrolysate formulas** (formulas with broken down proteins for easier digestion). Most babies will do great with a cow milk-based formula, which make up the majority of formulas available. A small percentage of babies may have a transient milk protein allergy—which usually presents with blood in the stool—and may require a protein hydrolysate formula. Because babies who are allergic to cow's milk are often allergic to soy milk as well, there is no medically compelling reason to use soy-based formulas.

Other options for babies include formulas enhanced by docosahexaenoic acid (DHA) and arachidonic acid (ARA) or formulas boosted with pre- and probiotics, but while there may be benefits to these additives, research has yet to clearly show consistent results. There are also formulas specially configured to assist with reflux, lactose intolerance, and fussiness—again, for the most part there is minimal data to support these benefits.

Often, parents will try several different types of formula before they feel like they have found the best fit—but bear in mind, it is probably more the maturation of the baby and their gut than the formula selection that makes the biggest difference. Any money saved on formula can go towards the baby's college fund—which is probably a better investment than purchasing the most expensive formula on the market, so don't be afraid to try generics! And of course, if there is any uncertainty as to which formula is best for your baby, talk to your pediatrician.

MILK PROTEIN ALLERGY

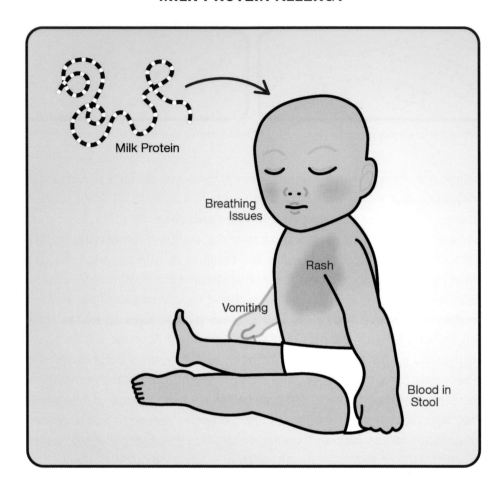

Milk protein allergies in children can be confusing, because there are a variety of different mechanisms which can cause a body to respond adversely to milk protein. Rarely, a baby can have a full blown allergic reaction to milk, with breathing issues, vomiting, and a pronounced rash; however, the more commonly seen problem is bleeding in the stool with or without associated fussiness.

Milk protein can irritate the lining of the intestinal tract, usually affecting the part closest to the anus. Although other foods can also cause irritation, such as egg and soy, cow's milk is by far the most common culprit. Because milk, soy, and egg proteins can pass through breast milk, both breastfed babies and formula-fed babies are equally affected.

Between 2–8 weeks of age, parents will start to notice visible blood in the stool, which may be accompanied by fussiness. In a breastfed child, the mother will need to eliminate all milk products from her diet, and possibly soy products as well (as there is often cross reactivity between the two proteins). If this does not work, the mother can try eliminating egg from the diet by itself or in addition to milk and soy.

For formula-fed babies, a switch to a **protein hydrolysate** formula should take care of the problem. These are formulas where the proteins are broken down so that the formula is easier to digest and will not irritate the intestines. Again, because of cross reactivity, soy formulas should not be utilized.

After making the necessary changes, babies should improve within three days. The vast majority of babies with milk protein allergies (the rectal bleeding type) will tolerate milk by their first birthday and about half will tolerate it by 6 months of age. A discussion with your pediatrician can help you figure out the best plan as to when and how to reintroduce milk back into your child's diet.

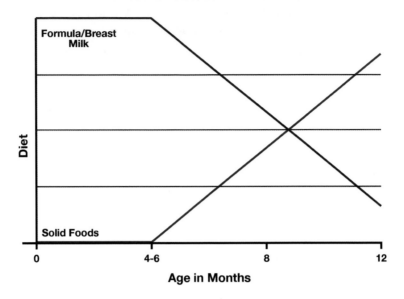

TRANSITIONING TO SOLIDS

Formula/Breast Milk

Diet

Solid Foods

0   4-6   8   12

Age in Months

This diagram is based on a 2001 World Health Organization report on complementary feeding.

Because infants begin their life on breast milk, parents often think that milk is essential for their child's diet even beyond the first year of life. But while milk is absolutely important for the first few months of life, once babies can start eating **solids**, the value of milk (breast, formula, or cow's) quickly diminishes. Milk's main purpose for humans (and animals) is to provide an easy source of nutrition to their babies until they are ready for solid foods—which offer a far greater diversity of nutrition. (Though milk does offer vitamin D and calcium, you can get plenty of vitamin D from the sun and all the calcium you need from meat, certain vegetables, soy, nuts, beans and other solid foods.)

By 1 year of age, the bulk of a child's nutrition should be from solid foods—ideally, they should be eating a well-balanced diet pulling from all of the food groups. At a maximum, a 1-year-old should be taking no more than 24 ounces of milk or formula, and as long as they are eating a balanced diet, there really is no minimum amount of milk that a 1-year-old needs.

Solid food introduction can begin anywhere between 4–6 months of age. Traditionally, parents in the United States start with cereal, move to fruits and vegetables, and add meats as the last food group. However, many experts now recommend reversing that order, as meats are the most nutritious in vitamins and minerals, and cereals are mostly filler foods with the least amount of nutrition. Regardless of the order, by 8–9 months of life at the latest, babies should be eating from every food group, the sooner the better.

Past concerns about causing food allergies led to a very conservative approach to introducing solid foods. Recommendations were to give only one new food every three days and certain foods such as peanuts and eggs were to be avoided until several years of age. New data has clearly shown that this thinking was incorrect and it is now known that early introduction of foods (particularly highly allergenic foods) is helpful and reduces the risk of food allergies in the future. Outside of honey (which can cause botulism), all other foods are safe to eat for babies as long as parents are careful of choking hazards.

As for the "one new food every three day rule," while this rule might help figure out what food caused an allergy by making the process of elimination easier, most kids with true allergies will have to undergo a series of tests if a true food allergy is suspected, making this rule unnecessary and a bit overly restrictive. It is perfectly reasonable and definitely easier to be aggressive and introduce several new foods at a time.

While there is a whole line of baby foods available at the supermarket, feel free to offer bite size portions of soft foods that parents eat for their own meals. Foods such as pastas, baked potatoes, soft meats, and steamed vegetables are all safe, nutritious, and tasty for babies to consume as soon as they can chew well. The more flavors children encounter early on, the less picky they will be later!

So go ahead and give them a bite of your dinner—they're probably eyeing you as you eat it and wondering where their portion is! As long as you can mash a food between your pointer finger and thumb, your baby can handle it; even with no teeth, baby's gums are powerful and can do more than you might think! The sooner they are eating real foods, the sooner you can cook one meal and make your life easier. Ultimately, if it is nutritious for you, it is nutritious for them.

So, how should you incorporate the solid foods into your current feeding schedule? The truth is there is no singular best way, but here is one method of doing it. Pick one meal to begin with, such as the feeding closest to breakfast time. Before giving formula or breast milk, start by allowing your baby to eat as much solid food as they will take. When they will no longer take any more solids, top them off with their normal bottle or breastfeed until they are full. Once they seem to have the hang of one meal, add a second around lunchtime, and soon thereafter a third around dinnertime. It is that simple!

Some simple rules of thumb with feeding:

1. **You are in charge of the quality of food; the child is in charge of the quantity of the food.** They will never shortchange themselves!

2. **Aim for a balanced diet over a week at a time.** Not every day and certainly not every meal needs to be perfectly balanced. It all goes to the same place!

3. **A child's growth controls their appetite, not the other way around.** Your kids will grow in spurts controlled by their hormones and appetite will follow accordingly. Again, they will never shortchange themselves!

Ideally, your child should be eating three solid food meals a day, covering all of the different food groups by 8–9 months of life. And by 1 year of age, children should essentially be eating what their parents are eating. The bottom line is there is a lot of freedom in how to start solids. Try lots of different foods and have some fun with it!

CHOKING RISKS

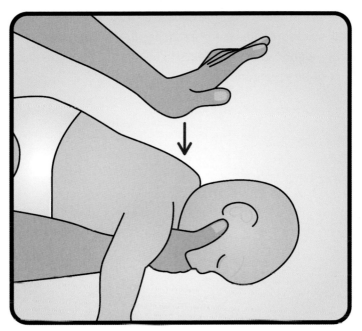

Place the infant stomach-down across your forearm and give five quick, forceful blows to the infant's back with the back of your hand.

As children begin solid foods, it is important for parents to be aware of **choking hazards**. Foods that are cylindrical, airway-sized, and compressible pose the highest risk of choking, as these types of food can wedge tightly into a child's airway and completely block it off.

The following are 10 foods that are commonly cited as posing a choking hazard:

1. Hot dogs
2. Peanuts
3. Carrots
4. Bone-in chicken
5. Candy

6. Meat
7. Popcorn
8. Fish with bones
9. Sunflower seeds
10. Apples

Obviously, it would be difficult—if not unreasonable—to completely avoid these foods. However, when children are eating the above foods, parents should be hypervigilant and may want to follow a few simple rules to be safer.

If eating a hot dog or similar food, cut it lengthwise before slicing it into pieces—coin shaped hot dog pieces can be dangerous. When cutting fruits and vegetables or similar food, cut them into quarters that are smaller than the child's airway. And finally, when selecting sweets for children, avoid ball shaped candies: for example, flat lollipops are safer than ball-shaped lollipops. And it is always a good idea for parents to become CPR-certified so that they will know what to do in the event of an emergency.

TAKE-HOME POINTS

★ Breast milk is the best food for babies during the first year of life; however, infant formula is an excellent alternative.

★ For the first few weeks of life, it is best to feed on-demand until the baby returns back to their birth weight.

★ After the infant returns to their birth weight, it is probably better for most families to move to a feeding schedule. This will help reduce fatigue and stress for parents.

★ Train your baby to feed during the day and sleep at night.

★ A well-fed baby will gain about ½–1 ounce of weight per day.

★ More than 60 percent of babies will spit-up, but as long as they are gaining weight and not excessively fussy there is little to worry about.

★ Parents are in charge of the quality of the food and the child is in charge of the quantity of the food.

★ The first few weeks of breastfeeding can be challenging, but it gets a lot easier after that.

★ Mothers should air out their nipples and use moisturizing creams to help prevent their nipples from getting tender.

★ Nipple confusion does not generally happen. Parents should feel comfortable using a pacifier to soothe babies and occasional bottle-feeds to reduce the burden on mom.

★ Breastfeeding is a "use it or lose it" endeavor, and when supply is an issue, pumping may help to stimulate more milk production.

★ In general, moms will do just fine for breastfeeding by following the same diet as they did for their pregnancy.

★ Breastfeeding moms should avoid smoking altogether and be judicious about their alcohol intake.

★ A good rule of thumb for storing breast milk is the "rule of 4": 4 hours at room temperature, 4 days in the refrigerator, or 4 months in the freezer.

★ The most common maternal medications that can cause problems with breastfeeding babies are sedatives taken for sleep, tranquilizing agents, mood-altering drugs, a few antibiotics, anti-tuberculosis medications, chemotherapeutic agents and seizure medications. Most other medications are safe, but it is always best to check with the pediatrician.

★ Never heat formula in the microwave as it can create pockets of hot formula that may burn the baby's mouth.

★ Most contraptions for bottle warming and cleaning are not necessary. Babies will be healthy and do just fine by following some sensible routines.

★ All formulas sold in the United States must meet the nutrient standard set by the Food and Drug Administration (FDA); as such, it is hard to go wrong with formula selection, whether it is a brand name with all the newest nutritional bells and whistles or a more cost-friendly generic brand.

★ A true milk protein allergy will cause babies to have bleeding in the stool, with or without associated fussiness. The vast majority of babies with milk protein allergies (the rectal bleeding type) will tolerate milk by their first birthday and about half will tolerate it by 6 months of age.

★ Aim for a balanced diet over a week at a time. Not every day—and certainly not every meal—needs to be perfectly balanced. It all goes to the same place!

★ A child's growth controls their appetite, not the other way around. Your kids will grow in spurts controlled by their hormones, and their appetite will follow accordingly. They will never shortchange themselves!

★ Ideally, your child should be eating three solid food meals a day covering all of the different food groups by 8–9 months of life. By 1 year of age, children should essentially be eating what their parents are eating.

★ Foods that are cylindrical, airway-sized, and compressible pose the highest risk of choking, as these types of food can wedge tightly into a child's airway and completely block it off.

What to Know Before Having Your Baby

Chapter 10

GOING OUT

ONCE YOU are settled into your feeding and sleeping routines, you will want to start going out with your baby to explore the world and all that it has to offer. It is around this time that new parents often become stressed, worrying about ultraviolet radiation and mosquito-borne diseases. By following some general tips, moms and dads can minimize environmental issues and enjoy traveling and the great outdoors with their new baby.

MOSQUITO REPELLENT

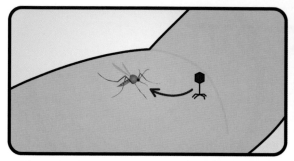

Mosquito biting an adult and ingesting a viral infection from the adult.

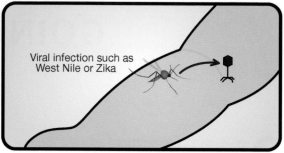

Mosquito biting a baby and transferring the viral infection.

Mosquitoes are not only a pest that people loathe, they are increasingly becoming a vector for diseases in the United States. As such, it is important to protect children from mosquito bites whenever possible by using **mosquito repellent**.

Below are some general rules of thumb when using mosquito repellent:

- Do not apply mosquito repellent to infants less than 2 months of age.

- Do not apply repellent over cuts or wounds.

- Do not apply to young children's hands, near the eyes, or near the mouth.

- For protection of child's face, apply repellent to adult hand and then rub gently onto their face.

- Do not apply under clothing.

- Dress children in light colored clothing that covers both their arms and legs.

- Avoid over-application. Use just enough to cover exposed skin and clothing.

- Repellent containing DEET (10–30 percent concentration) is safe for use on infants. Ten percent DEET is effective for up to 2 hours of protection and 30 percent DEET is effective for up to 6 hours of protection.

- Picardin is an effective synthetic alternative that provides protection for up to 2 hours.

- Oil of Lemon of Eucalyptus is an effective plant-based insect repellent that provides protection for up to 90 minutes, but do not use in children less than 3 years of age because of possible skin reactions.

What to Know Before Having Your Baby

- When needed, mosquito netting can be placed over bedding, strollers, and car seats for protection.

- After returning indoors, wash all treated skin with soap and water.

Mosquitoes need standing water to breed. To reduce the risk of mosquito bites, it is important to be vigilant about checking for standing water around the house. Listed below are some common sources of standing water that should be emptied at least once a week, if not more frequently:

- Bird baths

- Roof gutters

- Children's wading pools

- Flower pots

- Fire pits

SUNSCREEN

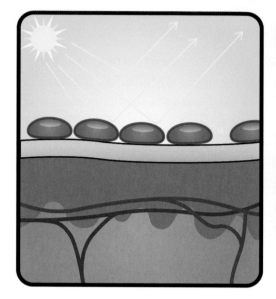

Physical sunscreens act by
reflecting the light.

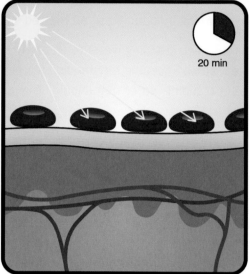

20 min

Chemical sunscreens act by
absorbing the light.

Sunscreen works by either blocking or absorbing harmful ultraviolet rays. Sunscreens that work by blocking UV rays are known as **physical sunscreens** or **inorganic sunscreens**, whereas the sunscreens that work by absorbing UV rays are known as **chemical sunscreens** or **organic sunscreens**.

Physical sunscreens, which tend to be thicker and greasier, contain either zinc oxide or titanium oxide and work by reflecting and scattering UV light rays. Chemical sunscreens are made up of complex organic molecules that work by absorbing the UV rays, which then undergo chemical reactions and release the energy as heat. Physical sunscreens work right away, but chemical sunscreens typically need to be applied 20 minutes before going out in the sun to achieve full protection.

Both types of sunscreens work well, and some sunscreens on the market contain both physical and chemical UV filters. Skin reactions can happen with either group of sunscreens but tend to happen more often with the chemical sunscreens. Trial and error will help to find the right sunscreen for each individual's skin type.

Some tips for sunscreen use:

• Use products with broad UVR (UVA and UVB) protection. To be safe, apply 20 minutes before sun exposure.

• SPF 15 or higher should always be used, although some experts recommend a minimum of SPF 30.

• Apply in appropriate amounts and reapply often (at least every 2 hours).

• Sunscreen safety requirements for babies under 6 months are not known. As such, babies under 6 months should be kept out of the direct sun. Use wide brimmed hats and loose-fit clothing to shield them. A small amount of sunscreen on exposed areas such as the face, hands, and feet when needed is probably safe and helpful.

• Limit time in the sun, especially during the peak sun hours (which are between the hours of 10 am and 2 pm.)

AIRPLANE TRAVEL

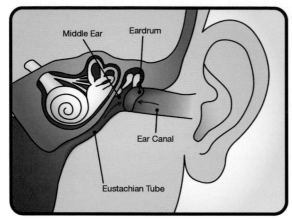

Equal Air Pressure

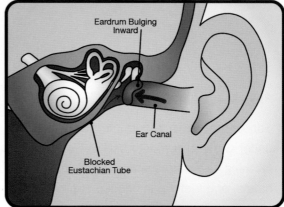

Unequal Air Pressure

Parents often worry about a baby's health when **traveling on an airplane** for the first time. Riding on an airplane poses no physical stress to the body that the baby cannot handle. The only problem may occur when taking off and landing—when the changing cabin pressure may cause some pain in the baby's ears. This can be alleviated by having the baby breastfeed or use a bottle or pacifier, which will help the middle ears to equilibrate by venting the Eustachian tube.

While there is no direct risk from the plane ride itself, the airport is full of germs and airplanes are crammed with people. But, as long as no one is touching the baby, there should be minimal exposure to germs. Ideally, travel on an airplane should happen after the first round of vaccines at 2 months of age, which also places the infant past the precarious 4–6 weeks mark for fever workups (see page 93). However, this is not a hard and fast rule, and when necessary babies can fly sooner.

Ultimately, like any other decision for the baby, risks and benefits should be weighed carefully with the input of the pediatrician.

TAKE-HOME POINTS

★ Parents can reduce the risk of mosquito-transmitted diseases by protecting their children with repellent and minimizing standing water around the home.

★ Sunscreen should offer broad UVR (UVA and UVB) protection, be a minimum of SPF 15–30, and be reapplied every 2 hours.

★ Airplanes are safe for babies, but look to minimize germ exposure by limiting the amount of people that touch them. Help alleviate cabin pressure changes in the ear by breastfeeding or using a bottle or pacifier. If possible, travel after the first round of vaccines at 2 months of age.

Conclusion

THE GOAL of writing this second book was mainly to give brand new parents who are going home with their first baby some peace of mind. There are so many little issues and concerns that come up those first few weeks, and if you have never seen them before, they can be quite vexing and angst producing.

This book is essentially a collection of all of the frequently asked questions I have encountered over the first 14 years of my career. Anything not covered in this book can of course be answered by your personal pediatrician.

I hope this book will give you some basic understanding of newborn concepts so that you can get more out of each check-up and visit. I also hope that reading this book has assuaged some of your early concerns so that you can enjoy your newborn baby to the fullest. It really is a precious time, and as everyone will tell you, it is fleeting!

About the Author

P ETER JUNG was born in Passaic, New Jersey in 1973, but has lived in Houston, Texas for most of his life. He eagerly followed his father's footsteps into pediatrics.

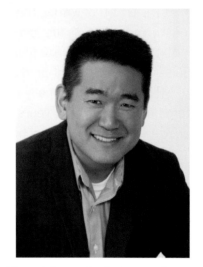

After receiving his board certification in pediatrics and becoming a Fellow of the American Academy of Pediatrics in 2002, Dr. Jung went into private practice with his father. When his father retired in 2004, Dr. Jung opened the doors to Blue Fish Pediatrics. Today, Blue Fish Pediatrics has grown to fourteen providers in three Houston-area locations.

Dr. Jung enjoys teaching pediatric residents, medical students, and nursing students at his community clinic year round. He has written for several local magazines, has been interviewed by local and national news programs about pediatric issues, and has taught several pediatric classes geared towards equipping parents.

Dr. Jung is active in his faith community at New Life Fellowship Church, where he leads the drama team and teaches the youth group. In his free time he enjoys basketball, softball, fishing, and spending time with his family.

About the Illustrator

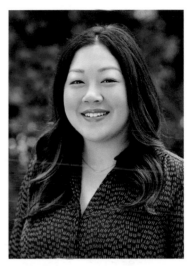

BECKY S. KIM has been doodling, drawing, and sketching on notebooks, menus, and napkins ever since she can remember. After getting her Bachelor of Arts in Visual Communication from American Intercontinental University, Becky utilized her degree in design by going into marketing, working in the restaurant/food industry for several years. She created websites, digital ads, menus and brochures for brands such as Popeye's, Fuddruckers and Pasta Prima. After a few years in administration, Becky returned to graphic design and worked for Woodlands Church, where her work was distributed on an international level, ranging from booklets to brochures to sermon series artwork. She was also the senior designer for Woodlands Seminary, which launched in January 2015. Currently, she works as an administrative assistant for commercial real estate and continues to do design as a freelancer.

In her free time, Becky loves to utilize her creative energies through cooking/baking, trying DIY home improvement projects, arts and crafts, and watercolor lettering. She enjoys trying new local restaurants, journaling, building furniture with her husband, and serving at her local church. Becky, her husband, and their dog currently live in Houston, Texas.

Becky enjoys painting, brush calligraphy, design, creating pretty things, DIY projects, building furniture, organizing, video games, cooking and eating. Becky, her husband and their dog currently live in Houston.

BLUE ✦ FISH
P E D I A T R I C S

Blue Fish Pediatrics is one of the fastest growing medical practices in Houston, Texas with 3 current locations and plans to add 2 new locations in the near future. After attending the same residency at Texas Children's Hospital and working in the same building but at different practices for 2 years, Drs. Jung and Pielop joined forces to open the first Blue Fish Pediatrics in 2005.

From its inception, the vision of Blue Fish Pediatrics has been to empower the caretaker of the child so that they can knowledgeably make medical decisions about their children with the help of our doctors. At each visit, our physicians endeavor not only to make the correct diagnosis and come up with the best treatment plan, but also strive to educate the family so that they understand what is happening with each illness their child encounters. It is the long-term relationships we build with each family that make our jobs fulfilling and fuel the growth of our practice. Learn more at www.bluefishmd.com.

Also by Peter Jung, M.D.

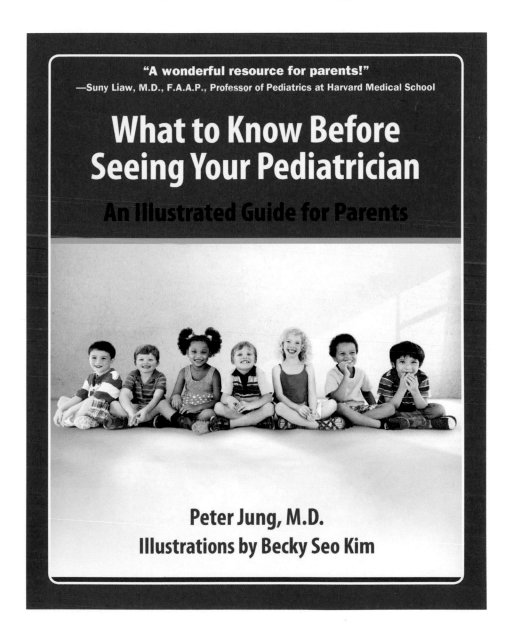

ISBN 978-1-57826-606-7

Available at www.hatherleighpress.com and wherever books are sold